You're Not a Caveman, Don't Eat Like One

You're Not a Caveman, Don't Eat Like One

Jennifer Swallow RD

ISBN: 0996504400
ISBN 13: 9780996504409
Library of Congress Control Number: 2015910068
Fit with Jen, Hanahan, SC
AKM 6-2

Contents

CHAPTER 1

You're Not a Caveman

You're not a caveman. As you climb into your SUV, charge your smartphone, listen to the radio, and drive to work, think of how your life is pretty much nothing like that of a caveman. Even if between the time this book is published and the time you start reading it, World War III suddenly annihilates modern technology and sends us back to the Stone Age, you're still not a caveman.

Why, then, would you eat like one? Are we meant to eat like our ancestors? Those are great questions. Let's follow that up with a few more: Are we meant to bathe every day? Wash our hands? Floss? Read? Fly an airplane? Drive a car? Travel into space? Leave Earth and voyage to the moon?

If older traditions were ultimately the best, then we would have no room for improvement. The backbone of civilization is agriculture. We would not have modern engineering, art, literature, and technology without agriculture. The Paleolithic diet was adequate for humans to survive in the Stone Age. *Survival* is the key word when considering what cavemen ate.

Before agriculture, eating plenty of meat was a way to consume sufficient calories when plant food was scarce. Cavemen could not be picky eaters, and their diets varied depending on the region and season. They did not have the luxury of entering a grocery store and selecting the optimal combination of imported foods to make healthy meals. They probably ate anything that they could find to fend off starvation. If they found something edible, they ate it, regardless of whether it was meat, grain, or legume. Their food was always what was in season and local but not necessarily ideal in terms of balanced nutrition.

Paleolithic humans were not restricted to one region of the world so their meals varied with each region they occupied. They undoubtedly experienced hard times and probably tried some very strange unsavory foods out of desperation. In fact, I doubt any cavemen thought, "Oh no, I can't eat this because it has gluten!" A much more likely thought was, "I need to eat this, or I will starve to death!"

We are no longer living in the Stone Age. Today, our diets contain too many calories, we get less physical activity, we have a longer lifespan, and we develop more chronic diseases. Most of us do not have to eat bugs or maggots to survive. We have a wide variety of imported and local options. And we generally don't have to fear being eaten by a wild animal. Now we need a diet that has some basis in our past roots, but one that is also *scientifically* proven to promote health and longevity.

The desire to lose weight has led some of us away from the standard American diet (SAD) and is also one reason that the Paleo diet continues to captivate countless minds. The Paleo trend is one of so many contemporary and past trends, such as the primal, Atkins, and ketogenic diets, touted for combating obesity.

New diets pop up so often that it is impossible to keep track of them all. Along with these diets, nutrition information expands and changes every day. For example, last week a reporter showed us how the cholesterol in eggs can increase the risk of heart disease. This week eggs are heralded in a news story as the best part of a nutritious breakfast. One minute experts are telling us to eat whole grains, and the next they show us why we should eat a gluten-free diet.

Amid the debate, one constant theme in the media is the battle between low-carb and low-fat diets. For every new low-carb diet, which is generally meat based, there is a new plant-based diet on the opposing side. To say the least, deciding what to eat can be frustrating.

A number of different diets are commonly championed as the healthiest, including the Paleo, Mediterranean, pescatarian, vegetarian, and vegan diets. The major differences are that Paleo is a meat-based diet, while the Mediterranean and vegetarian/vegan diets are plant based. (See "Brief Sample of Modern Diets" for foods excluded or included in popular diets.)

Brief Sample of Modern Diets

1. **Standard American Diet (SAD)**
   1. All foods allowed, with highly processed meats, salty, and sweet food preferred (heavy on soda, burgers, pizza, etc.)
2. **Atkins**
   2. Low carbohydrate, with a focus on dairy, meat, and eggs
3. **Paleo**
   3. No dairy, processed food, grains, or beans; focus on meat, eggs, fruits, and veggies (modeled after the diet of Paleolithic man)
4. **Mediterranean**
   4. Focus on veggies, fruit, fish, whole grains, olive oil, and beans; eat less meat/red meat
5. **Semivegetarian**
   5. No red meat (poultry, fish, eggs, and dairy allowed)
6. **Pescatarian**
   6. No poultry or red meat (fish, dairy, and eggs allowed)
7. **Lacto-ovovegetarian**
   7. No meat of any kind (dairy and eggs allowed)
8. **Lactovegetarian**
   8. No meat or eggs (dairy allowed)
9. **Strict Vegetarian/Vegan**
   9. No meat, eggs, or dairy (no animal products)

(Created by Jen Swallow from general knowledge/experience as a nutritionist.)

Diets one through three are meat based, while diets four through nine are plant based. So which one is the healthiest? Is it meat based or plant based? Low carb or high carb? Whole grains or gluten-free? How do we find the truth when we are bombarded with controversial nutrition information? We are constantly swimming in a sea of misinformation, and some of us feel as if we are drowning. Reaching the land of truth in this fast-paced age of Twitter, Facebook, and YouTube can be a daunting mission.

This book is dedicated to breaking down nutrition controversies and offering you the truth about fat, cholesterol, gluten, grains, beans, and the Paleo diet. I present facts about how your daily choices affect obesity and disease risk. If you want to eat a low-carb diet, that is your prerogative. I simply want you to know the difference between the fact and fiction of low-carb nutrition.

In many cultures, people often wish one another good health. We ask how family members are doing, hoping to hear everyone is in good health. Yet the most common conditions and diseases that plague Americans, such as obesity, hypertension, and heart disease, are preventable.[1–5] Some diseases can be more common for those with a relevant family history. Health can be influenced by good or bad genes, but genetics do *not* dictate health.[6–12]

The fat-mass-and-obesity-associated gene plays a role in obesity and type 2 diabetes.[13] Some people have one or two copies of this gene and are more likely to be overweight or obese than are people with no copies of the gene. But the type of food included in the diet can interact with these genes, which in turn makes obesity more or less likely in people who have the gene.[6–11] You can ultimately "turn on" or "turn off" some genes by changing your habits.

Governments have a responsibility to keep their citizens safe and allow them an opportunity for a healthy life, but good health is not a government-guaranteed right. Good health is largely a choice. It is a choice you make every day when you open your mouth, chew your food, and sip your beverages. Making the right choice can be easier when you know the whole truth about the consequences of that choice. My goal is to help arm you with the knowledge to make informed choices about your health. These choices might not only result in a body for the beach but also in a body and mind that can better stand up to the tests of time.

Real Nutrition Experts

One major reason why Americans are confused about which foods are healthy is the *source* of our nutrition information. Random celebrities or any Joe Schmo can write a weight-loss book and sell tons of copies despite a lack of relevant credentials or education. Taking diet advice from someone who does not have an in-depth understanding of nutrition can be risky.

What you put in your mouth may be *the* most important decision you make on a daily basis. Do you really want to put your health in the hands of someone who has little to no formal education in nutrition? On that note, let's examine the very idea of an expert in nutrition.

Which one do you consider an expert in nutrition?

- A caveman
- A reporter
- An acupuncturist
- An endurance runner
- An exercise science professor
- A registered and licensed dietitian nutritionist with a master's degree in nutrition

If you chose the last option, then this is the right book for you because it describes my credentials and education. Nutrition is my passion and my career. I am a registered dietitian and clinical nutritionist with a state license in dietetics and a background in personal training. In 2009, I became a personal trainer through the National Academy of Sports Medicine (NASM), and thereafter have worked with countless weight-loss clients.

My undergraduate degree from the University of Florida is in nutritional sciences. I completed a twelve-hundred-hour dietetic internship and subsequently graduated with a master's degree in nutrition. During my internship, I taught bariatric nutrition, diabetes, and weight-management classes to active-duty military and their dependents. Since then, I have given countless nutrition lectures, presentations, and grocery-store tours to a variety of audiences.

Seeing all of the controversial nutrition information available today can make anyone feel overwhelmed. Ask yourself some tough questions to get past this feeling. Who are you entrusting with your health? Would you seek out a hairdresser to design a house? Would you find a dentist to do your taxes? Would you ask an artist to develop a budget for your business? These scenarios seem ridiculous, but they are no more ridiculous than seeking nutrition advice from an aerospace engineer or a reporter.

The latest trendy diet book can be misleading as the average author doesn't even have a basic degree in nutrition, let alone an advanced degree, such as a master's or PhD in nutrition. Medical doctors are not required to have a degree in nutrition. Some take only one course in nutrition during their entire formal education. This does not make them a nutrition expert, which is why doctors often refer patients to professional nutritionists and dietitians for bariatric or diabetic nutrition education.

Yet so many patients believe that doctors are nutrition and weight-loss experts. This is simply not the case with most doctors. Visiting a doctor should be more about evaluating the type and seriousness of an illness and less about depending on the doctor to fix everything. Drugs and surgery can help with acute illnesses or injuries, such as bacterial infections or fractured bones. But they are not a cure for the top killer diseases, including heart disease and cancer.

Modern medicine is geared to manage disease once it occurs—not to prevent it. I see medicine in action regularly at my work with nursing home and rehab patients. An unhealthy lifestyle combined with obesity and drug abuse can destroy the body even at an early age. Before reading a medical history, I can already guess why people who are only fifty years old are admitted to the facility after having a heart attack or stroke. They are usually morbidly obese, sedentary, a long-time smoker, former smoker, or all of the above. My guesses turn out to be correct in most cases—a very sad truth, but a reality.

Unfortunately, most Americans are not educated in basic nutrition, especially when it comes to healthy eating. This makes them an easy target for misleading information. It is no wonder so many of us are overweight or obese!

Looking for proper guidance is important, but don't let this stop you from taking control of your own health. To achieve optimal health, your daily decisions should be based on several factors. First, use logic and common sense. Eating too many cheeseburgers—or any food—without enough physical activity to burn off the calories will make anyone fat. Next, read and research multiple credible scientific sources. Finally, always look up and review sources of information, even if the expert advice comes from those with relevant credentials. The moment you depend on someone else to make you feel healthy is the moment you have given up on your health.

I encourage you to think twice before taking advice from TV, magazines, and newspapers. The mass media are *not* credible scientific sources. Giving the public the whole truth is just not sensational enough for profit margins. Controversial half-truths, on the other hand, sell very well. Half-truths often come as sound bites on the news, offering only a tiny part of the information contained within complex nutrition studies. Don't base one of the most important decisions you make every day on some sensational headline on the evening news. Do your own research.

Please, Not Another Diet Book!

Science requires details, measurements, and a control to determine if an intervention does or does not work. All of these details are carefully recorded, whereas an anecdote told by a friend or neighbor can easily be recalled with errors. People are not perfect; they have trouble remembering what they ate yesterday, never mind the details of every meal for the past six months. This is why it is crucial to review multiple sources of reliable, science-based data before making a decision that will permanently affect your health.

I recently read several books about the modern version of the human Paleolithic diet and was disconcerted to see false or misleading information about grains, gluten, and beans. I was frustrated that well-respected people (albeit few with an advanced degree in nutrition) are propagating myths about beans, grains, and low-carb diets. I felt compelled to counter this misinformation with high quality facts. Thus was born the idea for *You're Not a Caveman, So Don't Eat Like One.*

Anyone can call himself or herself a *nutritionist*, even without relevant formal education, a college degree, or a true credential in nutrition. Some so-called nutritionists simply took a random test online to receive a certificate in the mail without passing any nutrition-related college-level courses. A *registered dietitian*, on the other hand, must have a college degree, a hands-on internship, and pass a national nutrition exam to obtain this credential.

This is vastly more nutrition-related education than most doctors receive in medical school.

Few other nutrition credentials exist that also require a college degree or graduate-level nutrition education. Dietitians, also known as registered dietitians and nutritionists (RDs or RDNs), are the ones actually hired to assess and advise sick patients about nutrition in hospitals and other health-care facilities. They are the only nutrition professionals most insurance companies reimburse for nutrition counseling on diabetes or weight loss.

My two degrees in nutrition, a state credential, and a national credential in nutrition will, I hope, give you a sense of security about the information that I provide. I work with doctors and nurses in a health-care facility. I assess and develop nutrition interventions for overweight, obese, underweight, and sick patients in a clinical setting. For years before my internship, I successfully coached weight-loss clients to improve their eating habits. I understand both the academic and practical aspects of nutrition.

Still, I encourage you to go beyond my opinions and anecdotes in the quest for quality diet and nutrition information. Because I always want you to feel secure about what you are learning, I only present information that is based on evidence. Many authors simply write diet-related stories or opinions sprinkled with a few studies; they sometimes make outrageous claims without any legitimate evidence. In this book, over three hundred scientific sources are cited.

Why have I taken the time to painstakingly support each idea with scientific evidence? My reason is certainly not to bore you to death with endless research studies. Finding one study—even a poorly designed study—to support an idea is very easy. Studies also seem to contradict one another because a ten-page research article is summarized into one sentence in a sensational news story. Nutrition studies are very complex, so they cannot be accurately summarized in a memorable sound bite.

Journalists and authors know the power of science. However, they often misuse cherry-picked studies and twist them into exciting stories for profit. They also tend to leave *specific* details out of general health claims, which can easily mislead the public. The breadth and quality of research in this book, therefore, is exceptional. I prefer to focus on the details rather than ignore them. Some full-length textbooks have fewer scientific references when compared with this book.

After reading several low-carb diet books, I was frustrated with the limited number or complete lack of scientific references. Even when the books had references, they were difficult to look up, not numbered, or not matched to a given statement. Some of their references were based on testimony or interviews.

When people want to know the truth about what affects their lives and health, it does them a disservice to offer questionable references or to present speculation as fact. Any college student who writes a research paper knows that TV, magazines, and Internet blogs are not credible sources. Stories are not science just as anecdotes and opinions are not facts.

After a steady stream of facts, I will offer you a detailed view into my own health, not out of ego, but simply as an example. I want you to see the practicality and experience based on my own life in addition to cold hard facts. For instance, the eating habits that I share at the end of this book have kept me thin and healthy for over eighteen years. We will explore how those habits have done the same for research participants around the world.

Ultimately, what you eat can make a major difference in the quality of your life. You have the freedom to eat anything you can afford. You can choose to eat steak or hot dogs every day. Any choices you make can be based on preferences, desires, or health. The choices you make, however, should not be based on misinformation or myths (even myths about cavemen).

Notes

1. "The American Heart Associations Diet and Lifestyle Recommendations", American Heart Association, Accessed March 16, 2015, http://www.heart.org/HEARTORG/GettingHealthy/NutritionCenter/HealthyEating/The-American-Heart-Associations-Diet-and-Lifestyle-Recommendations_UCM_305855_Article.jsp.
2. "The Health Effects of Overweight and Obesity", Centers for Disease Control and Prevention, Accessed February 9, 2015, http://www.cdc.gov/healthyweight/effects/index.html.
3. Min K. B., Min J. Y. "Android and gynoid fat percentages and serum lipid levels in United States adults." *Clin Endocrinol (Oxf)* May 29, 2014. [Epub ahead of print.]
4. Schwingshackl L., Dias S., Hoffmann G. "Impact of long-term lifestyle programmes on weight loss and cardiovascular risk factors in overweight/obese participants: a systemic review and network meta-analysis." *Syst Rev* 2014; 3 (1): 130.
5. Herbert J. R., Wirth M., Davis L., Davis B., Harmon B. E., Hurley T. G., et al. "C-reactive protein levels in African Americans: a diet

and lifestyle randomized community trial." *Am J Prev Med* 2013; 45 (4): 430–40.

6. Ornish D., Magbanua M. J., Weidner G., Weinberg V., Kemp C., Green C., et al. "Changes in prostate gene expression in men undergoing an intensive nutrition and lifestyle intervention." *Proc Natl Acad Sci* USA 2008; 105 (24): 8369–74.

7. Viguerie N., Montastier E., Maoret J. J., Roussel B., Corribes M., Valle C., et al. "Determinants of human adipose tissue gene expression: impact of diet, sex, metabolic status, and cis genetic regulation." *PLoS Genet* 2012; 8 (9): e1002959.

8. Remely M., Aumueller E., Jahn D., Hippe B., Brath H., Haslberger A. G. "Microbiota and epigenetic regulation of inflammatory mediators in type 2 diabetes and obesity." *Benef Microbes* 2014; 5 (1): 33–43.

9. Lourenco B. H., Qi L., Willett W. C., Cardoso M. A.; ACTION Study Team. "FTO genotype, vitamin D status, and weight gain during childhood." *Diabetes* 2014; 63 (2): 808–14.

10. Qi Q., Chu A. Y., Kang J. H., Huang J., Rose L. M., Jensen M. K., et al. "Fried food consumption, genetic risk, and body mass index: gene-diet interaction analysis in three US cohort studies." *BMJ* 2014; 348: g1610.

11. Qi Q., Li Y., Chomistek A. K., Kang J. H., Curhan G. C., Pasquale L. R., et al. "Television watching, leisure time physical activity, and the genetic predisposition in relation to body mass index in women and men." *Circulation* 2012; 126 (15): 1821–27.

12. "Genetics Home Reference: Your Guide to Understanding Genetic Conditions, Mutations and Health", Accessed April 4, 2015, http://ghr.nlm.nih.gov/handbook/mutationsanddisorders/predisposition.

13. "Genetics Home Reference: Your Guide to Understanding Genetic Conditions, Genes > FTO", Accessed April 4, 2015, http://ghr.nlm.nih.gov/gene/FTO.

CHAPTER 2

Nutrition Controversy

Our Paleolithic ancestors were regularly on the move in search of shelter or food because they could not hop into a car, pull up to a drive-through window, and order a burger. Caveman were far more active than modern humans.

Today we barely have to lift a finger to order fast food and have it delivered to us as we sit and watch TV for an entire evening. The foods we eat now are very different from what cavemen ate in the Stone Age—and they are affecting us in ways that we are just beginning to understand.

Thanks in part to our diet, more than one out of every three children in the United States are overweight or obese. Over the past thirty years, obesity has doubled in children and quadrupled in teens.[1] Severely obese teens are commonly afflicted with diabetes, high blood pressure, high cholesterol, and inflammation.[2] These are just some ways in which the standard American diet (SAD)—characterized by highly processed and packaged foods like soda, candy, ice cream, fries, hot dogs, and pizza—wreaks havoc on long-term health.

These are the very same foods that I once enjoyed eating on a regular basis. There was plenty of cholesterol and fat in each meal, starting with bacon and eggs for breakfast, a cheeseburger for lunch, and fried chicken for dinner. This kind of diet can lead to obesity, hypertension, heart disease, diabetes, and kidney failure.[1-9]

Hypertension, also known as high blood pressure, can lead to kidney failure, heart attack, or stroke.[10, 11] Hypertension is on nearly every medical history I see as a clinical nutritionist. Diabetes can also destroy kidneys, cause pain in the limbs, and require leg amputation, which I see often in older patients. The fast-food-loving, TV-addicted American lifestyle is to blame. The bottom line is that SAD combined with inactivity can make us fat and sick. This is a problem that is wrecking our health and burdening our economy.

Most experts know that SAD is unhealthy, so what is the alternative? We need to embrace a dependable long-term solution. Unfortunately, there is still a great deal of controversy about which diet is best. A meat-centered caveman-style diet, however, has dominated many other popular options despite its emphasis on high-fat or high-cholesterol foods such as red meat and eggs. Long-term evidence to support the health benefits of this fad is minimal at best.

Why the Paleo Diet?

The Paleo diet has spread a fear of gluten and grains around the globe. This trend has proven to be highly contagious with gluten-free labels adorning the aisles of grocery stores, supermarkets, corner stores, and some restaurants. Many of my friends and family members have turned to the Paleo diet to lose weight.

Atkins, the Zone, primal, and the ketogenic diets have also led some Americans to ditch gluten and carbs in general. Some low-carb diets that permit only 5 or 10% carbs are extreme because of how much cheese, bacon, sausage, and butter are encouraged on these diets. Why would I then choose to criticize Paleo? Why not focus on the more extreme Atkins diet or the ketogenic diet? While a number of low-carb diets have been trendy for many years, the Paleo diet, in particular, has taken over the spotlight.

As I write this book, a new meet-up group called Living Paleo, Charleston, posted its first event for the year.[12] If you are familiar with the popular online community called Reddit, you might know that the Paleo Reddit community has over 75,000 subscribers compared with 260 for Atkins, 700 for primal, and 3,000 for low-carb subscribers.[13]

The premise of the modern Paleo diet is to eat meat, fruits, and vegetables like cavemen ate during the Paleolithic era. Beans and grains are not Paleo friendly because cavemen presumably did not eat them. Many redeemable aspects of the diet attract even skeptical consumers. For instance, a few positive Paleo principles include focusing on fruits and vegetables, avoiding sugary treats, avoiding dairy (though butter is in many Paleo recipes), and reducing highly processed foods. Undoubtedly every diet should include fresh fruits and vegetables. Regardless of these positive features, numerous myths have been propagated by Paleo supporters about dietary fat, gluten, grains, and beans. But this book is not about analyzing or verifying the original caveman diet. Rather, it is about highlighting new and current diet facts supported by modern research.

What Is Gluten?

Gluten is a protein found in many grains such as wheat, barley, and rye.[15] It is commonly blamed for obesity, inflammation, and inflammatory diseases. It is found in anything that has wheat flour, including bread, tortillas, pasta, cookies, and cake. Obviously, cookies and cake are easy to overeat, making them common contributors to obesity. Gluten, however, is not the only ingredient in cookies and cake, which also contain added fat and sugar.

Which foods truly make us fat? Is gluten truly to blame? Refined and processed white grains are fittingly left out of Paleo meal plans, but fiber-rich whole grains are also rejected. Inevitably, this leads to eating more animal products, such as beef, chicken, eggs, and butter, because they have no carbs. Society has come to believe that meat and eggs are essential to a healthy diet. Taking this a step further, Paleo followers have somehow even redeemed bacon and relabeled it as a health food.

Popular Paleo recipes feature bacon or butter. Saturated fat is supposedly harmless and immaterial to weight loss. Paleo experts, in general, often embrace dietary fat. Is bacon healthier than gluten? Where is the evidence proving that gluten is bad and bacon is good for our health?

Junk foods that contain gluten—such as cake, cookies, and donuts—are definitely unhealthy. But all of these foods also contain fat in the form of oil or butter. Shredded wheat, bran flakes, and puffed wheat all contain gluten as well, but are they as unhealthy as cake and cookies? The following chapters will review the current evidence about the effects of gluten, bacon, low-carb diets, and chronic disease.

Low-Carb Diets

The Paleo diet is an alleged cure-all for obesity, diabetes, and other chronic diseases. Perhaps this is because, at first glance, the diet appears healthier than others. No limit is set on the total amount of carbs in theory, but this amount ends up much lower in practice. Grains and grain-based foods are the main contributors to carb intake, so when these foods are cut out, the total carb intake tends to drop.

Low-carb agendas have long advised us about the evils of sugar, bread, and rice. There are many differences between Paleo and Atkins, for example, but they both promote one key principle: increasing protein and fat intake at the expense of carb intake. The rationale is that carbs, especially grains and gluten-based foods, supposedly make us fat and cause chronic diseases.[14, 15] Eating more fat and protein, on the other hand, can put the body in "fat-burning" mode. For this reason, low-carb pundits often criticize the low-fat diet and even suggest that Americans are eating a low-fat diet.

Big Fat Myths

Renewed popularity of bacon and butter has ignited mass confusion about saturated fat. We have known for quite some time that these foods can clog the arteries, so why the sudden change? Is saturated fat harmless? Was the fear of bacon all based on lies? Do Americans now eat a low-fat diet with no resolution of any health problems?

Many low-carb fans believe that one man is responsible for the big "fat fraud." Ancel Keys, a scientist who published some data on the link between dietary fats and heart disease over fifty years ago, has been criticized by low-carb and Paleo pundits.[16] Keys is blamed for misleading the public into a fat-hating frenzy. He is credited with supposedly leading Americans to eat a low-fat diet, which has not made a dent in the rise of obesity, heart disease, or diabetes.

The story goes like this: "We are eating a low-fat and low-cholesterol diet, yet we are still fat and sick. Therefore, saturated fat must be harmless." In this chapter, let's delve into these questions: Do Americans really eat a low-fat diet? Is Ancel Keys responsible for making Americans hate fat? The next chapter tackles the claim that saturated fat intake is harmless to human health.

The term "low-fat diet" generally means less than 30% of total daily calories are from fat, but it has no other specific standard.[17, 18] It's a vague term that can easily mislead people. A low-fat diet can be 29% or 15% or 5% of total calories from fat, which can be any kind of fat with no set proportion of saturated (bad fat) or monounsaturated or polyunsaturated (good fats).

Keys's research findings did not result in more Americans eating a low-fat diet. On the contrary, Americans love fat! When you go to a fast-food restaurant and see people ordering a bacon double cheeseburger with fries, do you think to yourself, "Wow that is so low in fat!" Probably not. Whether you visit a BBQ restaurant with ribs, a pizza place with meat-lovers deep dish, or a steakhouse with a giant fried onion, it's clear what kind of food Americans like.

Americans do *not* eat a low-fat or a low-cholesterol diet.[19] If anything, the American diet is moderate in fat (34%) and similar to the average diet in other developed countries, such as Ireland (35% fat), Sweden (36% fat), Finland (33%), and France (36%).[20–24] In fact, populations in many other countries around the world, such as China and Japan, eat less fat than we do.[19, 24, 25]

Do Americans follow government dietary recommendations? *The Dietary Guidelines for Americans 2010* suggests eating less than 10% of calories from saturated fat, out of 20–35% total fat, and less than 300 mg of cholesterol.[26] The average American commonly meets these guidelines for saturated fat and cholesterol, though men tend to surpass them or reach the maximum end of the guidelines.[19] The Paleo diet suggests 40% of calories from fat.[27] Vegetarians and vegans are two populations of Americans who eat less total fat and less saturated fat.[28] The average vegan eats half of the recommended amounts of saturated fat and zero cholesterol.[28]

Fat Conclusion

Low-carb diets are higher in fat than the regular American diet and even more so when compared with plant-based diets.[19, 27, 28] Here is the ranking from highest-fat to lowest-fat diet: the Paleo, average American, vegetarian, and vegan diets.[19, 27, 28] Vegans usually eat from 25 to 28% of their calories from fat. The average plant-based diet is rich in carbs and fiber with much less fat than the Paleo diet or American diet.[19, 27, 28] Several doctors and researchers have used a very low-fat, whole-food vegan diet with only 10% fat to successfully treat heart disease, cancer, and diabetes.[29-32] This type of diet is drastically different from the average US diet. Cutting the average fat intake down to half or one third of one's usual intake should be considered a "low-fat diet," not simply reducing it by 5%.

Percent of Nutrients in Different Diets

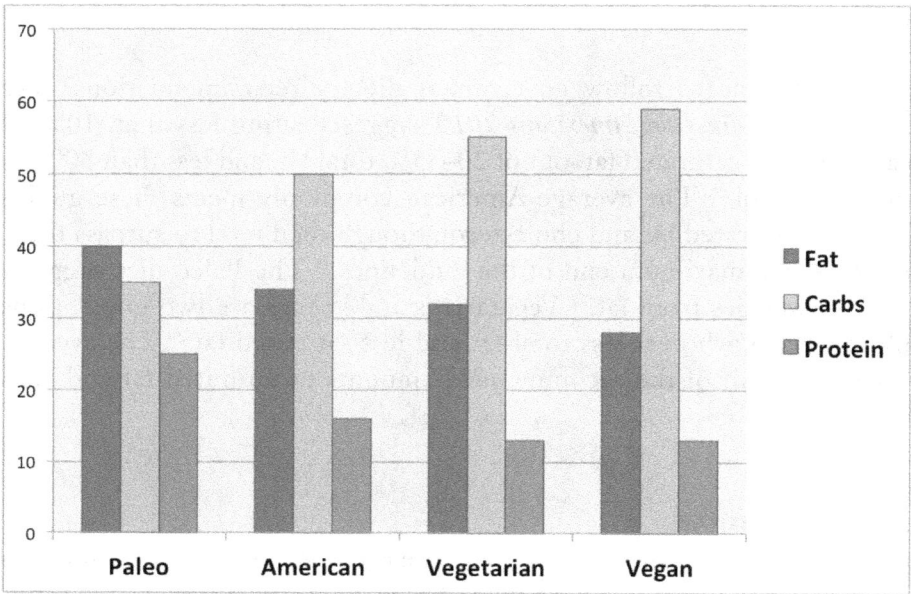

(Vegetarian and vegan diets are plant-based diets. The vegetarian diet excludes meat, while the vegan diet excludes dairy, eggs, and meat.)

In the past, fat consumption was a bit higher, by about 6%,[25] than it is today, but that does not mean Americans eat a low-fat diet. We managed to replace some of those calories with processed carbs, such as soda. Fat consumption is now moderate and similar to that of other developed countries. The modern American diet has not improved because one unhealthy food was simply swapped for another. We cannot focus excessively on the quantity of fat or carbs to improve the quality of our diets. Healthy eating should be about eating healthy foods without a strict goal for carb or fat intake. Numbers are important, but the type of food included in the diet is at least equally important.

Notes

1. "Childhood Obesity Facts", Centers for Disease Control and Prevention, Accessed March 4, 2015, http://www.cdc.gov/healthyyouth/obesity/facts.htm.
2. Michalsky M. P., Inge T. H., Simmons M., Jenkins T. M., Buncher R., Helmrath M., et al. "Cardiovascular risk factors in severely obese adolescents: The Teen Longitudinal Assessment of Bariatric Surgery (Teen-LABS) Study." *JAMA Pediatr*; Mar 2 2015.
3. Ledikwe J. H., Smiciklas-Wright H., Mitchell D. C., Miller C. K., Jensen G. L. "Dietary patterns of rural older adults are associated with weight and nutritional status." *J Am Geriatr Soc* 2004; 52 (4): 589–95.
4. Sun J., Buys N. J., Hills A. P. "Dietary pattern and its association with the prevalence of obesity, hypertension and other cardiovascular risk factors among Chinese older adults." *Int J Environ Res Public Health* 2014; 11 (4): 3956–71.
5. Davis J. N., Hodges V. A., Gillham M. B. "Normal-weight adults consume more fiber and fruit than their age- and height-matched overweight/obese counterparts." *J Am Diet Assoc* 2006; 106 (6): 833–40.
6. Brown C. D., Higgins M., Donato K. A., Rohde F. C., Garrison R., Obarzanek E., et al. "Body mass index and the prevalence of hypertension and dyslipidemia." *Obes Res* 2000; 8 (9): 605–19.
7. Tuso P., Stoll S. R., Li W. W. A plant-based diet, atherogenesis, and coronary artery disease prevention. *Perm J* 2015; 19 (1): 62–7.
8. Buttar H. S., Li T., Ravi N. "Prevention of cardiovascular disease: role of exercise, dietary interventions, obesity and smoking cessation." *Exp Clin Cardiol* 2005; 10 (4): 229–49.
9. Banerjee T., Crews D. C., Wesson D. E., Tilea A. M., Saran R., Rios-Burrows N., et al. "High dietary acid load predicts ESRD among adults with CKD." *J Am Soc Nephrol* 2015. [Epub ahead of print.]

10. Botdorf J., Chaudhary K., Whaley-Connell A. "Hypertension in cardiovascular and kidney disease." *Cardiorenal Med* 2011; 1 (3): 183–92.

11. "High Blood Pressure", National Institutes of Health; Medline Plus, Accessed Nov 15, 2014, http://www.nlm.nih.gov/medlineplus/ency/article/000468.htm.

12. "Living Paleo Charleston", Accessed February 1, 2015, http://www.meetup.com/Living-Paleo-Charleston/events/220225414/.

13. "Reddit", Accessed February 1, 2015, https://www.reddit.com/.

14. "Cut Down on Carbs to Reduce Body Fat", Mercola.com, Accessed March 17, 2015, http://articles.mercola.com/sites/articles/archive/2011/07/08/cut-down-on-carbs-to-reduce-body-fat.aspx.

15. Biesiekierski J. R., Muir J. G., Gibson P. R. "Is gluten a cause of gastrointestinal symptoms in people without celiac disease?" *Curr Allergy Asthma Rep* 2013; 13 (6): 631–38.

16. "The Fear of Saturated Fat and Cholesterol", Sébastien Noël, Accessed February 25, 2015, http://paleoleap.com/fear-of-saturated-fat-and-cholesterol/.

17. Lecheminent J. D., Gibson C. A., Sullivan D. K., Hall S., Washburn R., Vernon M. C., et al. "Comparison of a low carbohydrate and low fat diet for weight maintenance in overweight or obese adults enrolled in a clinical weight management program." *Nutr J* 2007; 6: 36.

18. Bueno N. B., de Melo I. S., de Oliveira S. L., da Rocha Ataide T. "Very-low-carbohydrate ketogenic diet v. low-fat diet for long-term weight loss: a meta-analysis of randomized controlled trials." *Br J Nutr* 2013; 110 (7): 1178–87.

19. "What We Eat in America 2011–2012", USDA Food Surveys, Accessed September 5, 2015, http://ars.usda.gov/Services/docs.htm?docid=13793.

20. Harrington K. E., McGowan M. J., Kiely M., Robson P. J., Livingstone M. B., Morrissey P. A., Gibney M. J. "Macronutrient intakes and food sources in Irish adults: findings of the North/South Ireland Food Consumption Survey." *Public Health Nutr* 2001; 4 (5A): 1051–60.

21. Becker W. "Dietary guidelines and patterns of food and nutrient intake in Sweden." *Br Nutr* 1999; 81 Suppl 2: S113–17.

22. Jost J. P., Simon C., Nuttens M. C., Bingham A., Ruidavets J. B., Cambou J. P., et al. "Comparison of dietary patterns between population samples in the three French MONICA nutritional surveys." *Epidemiol Sante Publique* 1990; 38 (5–6): 517–23.

23. Pietinen P., Paturi M., Reinivuo H., Tapanainen H., Valsta L. M. "FINDIET 2007 Survey: energy and nutrient intakes." *Public Health Nutr* 2010; 13 (6A): 920–24.

24. Zhou B. E., Stamler J., Dennis B., Moag-Stahlberg A., Okuda N., Robertson C., et al. "Nutrient intakes of middle-aged men and women in China, Japan, United Kingdom, and United States in the late 1990s: the INTERMAP study." *Hum Hypertens* 2003; 17 (9): 623–30.

25. Willcox D. C., Willcox B. J., Todoriki H., Suzuki M. "The Okinawan diet: health implications of a low-calorie, nutrient-dense, antioxidant-rich dietary pattern low in glycemic load." *J Am Coll Nutr* 2009; 28 Suppl: 500s–516s.

26. "Dietary Guidelines for Americans 2010", Office of Disease Prevention and Health Promotion, Accessed March 17, 2015, http://www.health.gov/dietaryguidelines/2010.asp.

27. "The Paleo Diet Premise," Loren Cordain, The Paleo Diet, Accessed February 10, 2015, http://thepaleodiet.com/the-paleo-diet-premise.

28. Rizzo N. S., Jaceldo-Siegl K., Sabate J., Fraser G. E. "Nutrient profiles of vegetarian and nonvegetarian dietary patterns." *J Acad Nutr Diet* 2013; 113 (12): 1610–19.

29. McDougall J., Thomas L. E., McDougall C., Moloney G., Saul B., Finnell J. S., Richardson K., Peterson K. M. "Effects of 7 days on an ad libitum low-fat vegan diet: the McDougall Program cohort." *Nutr J* 2014; 13 (1): 99.

30. Barnard N. D., Cohen J., Jenkins D. J., Turner-McGrievy G., Gloede L., Green A., Ferdowsian H. "A low-fat vegan diet and a conventional diabetes diet in the treatment of type 2 diabetes: a randomized, controlled, 74-wk clinical trial." *Am J Clin Nutr* 2009; 89 (5): 1588S–1596S.

31. Dewell A., Weidner G., Sumner M. D., Chi C. S., Ornish D. "A very-low-fat vegan diet increases intake of protective dietary factors and decreases intake of pathogenic dietary factors." *J Am Diet Assoc* 2008; 108 (2): 347–56.

32. Frattaroli J., Weidner G., Dnistrian A. M., Kemp C., Daubenmier J. J., Marlin R. O., Crutchfield L., Yglecias L., Carroll P. R., Ornish D. "Clinical events in prostate cancer lifestyle trial: results from two years of follow-up." *Urology* 2008; 72 (6): 1319–23.

CHAPTER 3

Low Carb or
Low Fat?

Low-carb diets have been popular for many years. After comparing the average carb/fat intake of omnivores to vegans, you might wonder whether a low-carb or Paleo diet is as effective or more effective for weight loss.

There is a huge difference between a 5% fat diet and a 29% fat diet. And studies don't evaluate the difference between fats from refined foods like oil and margarine versus whole natural foods like avocado and walnuts. [1-3] To determine if a specific food is healthy, the *type* of fat must be defined and not just the *amount* of fat in it. The following items are low-fat and high-carb foods: soda, candy, beans, sugar, and figs. Obviously, some low-fat foods are very healthy and some are junk. One low-fat diet can be based on soda, candy, and white bread, while another can be based on a combination of fruits, vegetables, beans, and whole grains. Do these two low-fat diets sound equally healthy? Using the term "low-fat" to describe a food or even a diet does not tell us whether it is healthy or natural.

Many scientific studies have compared the two diets with mixed results.[3-15] In the last chapter, we saw how eating fat can hurt weight-loss efforts, but what about when carbs are minimized? American vegans tend to eat a high-carb diet, yet they are the leanest of them all. So this disproves the low-carb propaganda. Vegans eat about 60% carbs on average, which is more than the regular American diet, while the Paleo diet is around 40% carbs.[1, 2]

Low-carb diets are still commonly used for weight loss. Some short-term studies demonstrate that participants can lose more weight on a low-carb diet than on a low-fat diet.[3–10] Other studies demonstrate that low fat is equally effective.[11, 13, 14] Why does one study contradict the next?

There are many reasons why diet studies contradict one another:

- There are no standard definitions of the terms "low fat" or "low carb."
- There are no rules for the type of fat or type of carbs allowed in either diet.
- Most studies are too short in duration for practical results.

Defining Low Fat and Low Carb

Diet studies are inconsistent in defining the terms "low carb" and "low fat." As previously mentioned, the low-fat diet can be anything less than 30% of total calories from fat or in some cases right around 30% fat, which is very close to SAD at 34% fat. So you can be considered as eating a low-fat diet by simply reducing your fat intake by 4%. This level of fat should really be considered *moderate* and not low, which means that most low-fat studies are not examining a diet low in fat. Such studies are merely looking at a control diet with trivial changes.

Low-carb diets, on the other hand, usually include less than 10% of total calories from carbs, which is radically different from SAD at 50% carbs. This means that people are not lowering their carb intake by 4% or even cutting it in half; they are actually reducing it by 80%. To top it all off, many of these studies do not count calories or keep a log of what the subjects are actually eating.

Does it seem logical to compare one diet that is close to average with a diet that is radically different?

If we compared a 5% fat diet with a 5% carb diet, then we might see similar weight-loss results, but such restrictions are not necessary for normal people. Radical changes like these are very difficult to stick with when people are already accustomed to a moderate ratio of nutrients.

Let's take a look at the results of several low-carb diet studies. After reviewing the following table, you might come to the conclusion that low-carb diets are indeed more effective than low-fat diets for weight loss.[3-10] In a short period of six months or less, a very low-carb diet, such as Atkins or ketogenic, can result in a weight loss of up to 26 lb.[7] This is equal to losing about 1 lb per week. As subjects continue the diet for more than twelve months, however, results are less consistent and less dramatic.[11-15] At the two-year mark, some low-carb dieters lost only 10 lb and some lost 15 lb,[14, 15] which is due to partial weight regain.

Low-Carb and Low-Fat Diets

Year	Author	Subjects	Length	Low carb	Low fat	Results
2014	Rhyu et al[3]	20 (athletes)	3 wk	4% carbs	30% fat	Low carb= -8 lb, low fat= -3 lb
2005	Nickols-Richardson et al[4]	28	1.5 mo	Atkins-based	22% fat	Low carb= -14 lb, low fat= -9 lb
2007	Halyburten et al[5]	93	2 mo	4% carbs	30% fat	Low carb= -17 lb, low fat= -14 lb
2006	Daly et al[6]	102	3 mo	34% carbs	33% fat	Low carb= -8 lb, low fat= -9 lb
2007	Tay et al[7]	88	6 mo	4% carbs	30% fat	Low carb= -26 lb, low fat= -22 lb
2011	Summer et al[8]	81	6 mo	Atkins-based	30% fat	Low carb= -20 lb, low fat= -11 lb
2003	Mueller-Cunningham et al[9]	54	6 mo	No control	11% fat	Low fat= -13 lb
2010	Krebs et al[10]	33	9 mo	<20 g carbs	<30% fat	Low carb= -29 lb, low fat= -16 lb
2009	Brinkworth et al[11]	106	1 yr	40 g carbs	30% fat	Low carb= -30 lb, low fat= -30 lb (both=1400-1600 calories)
2008	Alhassan et al[12]	181	1 yr	Atkins	10% fat Ornish	Low carb= -18 lb, low fat= -14 lb
2005	Dansinger et al[13]	93	1 yr	Atkins	10% fat Ornish	Low carb= -5 lb, low fat= -7 lb
2010	Foster et al[14]	307	2 yr	Atkins	30% fat	Low carb= -15 lb, low fat= -15 lb
2008	Shai et al[15]	322	2 yr	Atkins-based	30% fat AHA-based	Low carb= -10 lb, low fat= -6 lb

Where Does Paleo Stand?

The modern Paleo diet was not originally intended to be a very low-carb diet, yet in real life it is. Some Paleo dieters feel that they do not eat a low-carb diet because there is no set limit to how many grams of carbs they can eat. The modern Paleo diet, according to the website of author and Paleo expert Dr. Loren Cordain, should be 19–35% protein and 35–45% carbs.[2] This leaves a range between 20 and 46% of calories from fat. These wide ranges allow a lot of room for variation. The site also suggests that over half of total calories should come from meat.[2]

One might think that the Paleo diet would even out and land somewhere in the middle of these ranges; after all, meals are combined each day, but this is simply not the case with the practical version of this diet. Within four Paleo recipes for different meals, the average amount of carbs is about 10% of total calories, which leaves 30% protein and 60% fat.[16–18] Even if the carb intake is doubled by adding more fruit or veggies, this still leaves a carb intake of about 20%.

The only way that strict Paleo dieters can achieve more than 10 or 15% of calories from carbs would be to eat over six cups of cooked veggies and/or fruits daily.[19] Raw vegetables like spinach or lettuce are low in calories and very low in carbohydrates.[19] One cup of raw spinach only has 1 g of carbohydrate, while cooked spinach has 7 g.[19]

Eating six cups of cooked spinach equals 42 g of carbs, which comes out to 11% of calories in a 1,500-calorie diet. The same amount of strawberries comes out to 66 g of carbs, which is 17% carbs in the same type of diet. Eating six cups of fruit is less likely than eating six cups of veggies since most Paleo recipes are based on meat and veggies. If you double those numbers and eat twelve cups of cooked veggies a day, only about 25% of calories would come from carbs, which still means that carbs are cut in half when compared to the average American diet.

Compare spinach with a cup of oatmeal that contains 30 g of carbs and you can see how it would be difficult to reach more than 20% carbs without grains. Beans are also very high in complex carbs and low in fat.[19] So cutting whole grains and beans out of a diet, not to mention all processed foods, can make it virtually impossible to eat a regular amount of carbs. This means a low-carb diet is basically inevitable without these foods. Starchy vegetables like potatoes are high in carbs, but they are usually discouraged on the Paleo diet. See the table below for carbs per cup of different foods.

Carbohydrate Grams per Cup of Food

Carbs per Cup (g)

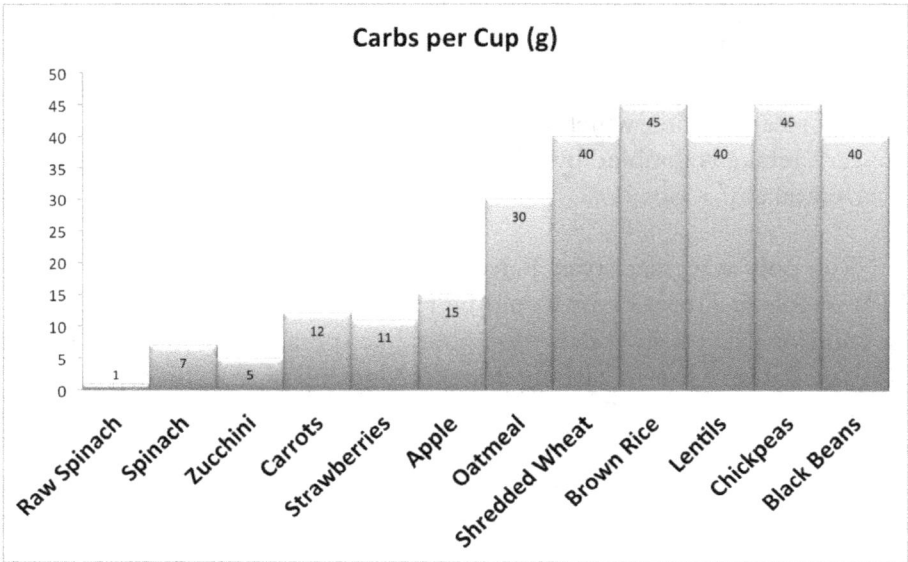

Data compiled by Jen Swallow from US Department of Agriculture, Agricultural Research Service. 2014. USDA National Nutrient Database for Standard Reference, Release 27. Nutrient Data Laboratory home page, http://www.ars.usda.gov/nutrientdata.

The Paleo diet is in practice a high-fat and low-carb diet as most Paleo recipes are very low in carbs. People who try this diet seem to have their own version: some do not eat dairy, some add butter, some eat gluten-free grains, and some eat unlimited bacon. A strict Paleo diet does not include any dairy, grains, or beans. Compliance can be a struggle for dieters. Keeping the conditions in diet studies constant is very difficult, and this is one of many reasons why results can contradict one another. The Paleo diet is no exception to this general phenomenon.

The reality is that low-carb diets work *temporarily*. First, most subjects are more compliant upon starting a diet and less compliant after six months. The body will always crave carbs because they are the preferred source of energy for the brain and other tissue. Second, writing down what we eat is tedious, and we often forget how much or what exactly we ate.

Research on the human diet is extremely difficult and expensive because of all the factors that affect what we eat.

Nutrition research conclusions are often inconsistent because people are so inconsistent with what they eat and how much they exercise. Just try writing down the amount and type of foods you eat every day. This, along with timing your workouts and keeping a log of exercises, can become a tedious task. Add in the effects of genes, age, smoking, and alcohol intake, and it becomes increasingly clear how many factors can affect weight loss. Diet cannot truly be examined in the absence of everything else that affects health. But it can be estimated and controlled for in well-designed studies.

Type of Fat or Carb

The specific type of fats or carbs consumed in diet studies is almost never described. In the world of nutrition, there are many different types of fat, including essential, nonessential, short-chain, and long-chain fatty acids. Some fats are healthy and some are not. For example, omega-3 fats are healthy and essential, but saturated fat is not essential and can be unhealthy in large amounts.[20]

Regardless of whether we count fat, protein, or carb grams, daily food intake is not consistently tracked in most studies, so estimating what and how much subjects eat is rarely done with accuracy. Researchers sometimes include monthly questionnaires or a scheduled twenty-four-hour recall, but daily food choices are not usually logged. Even if each meal were recorded, some low-fat diets are healthy and some are not, which could make a world of difference in terms of weight loss.

A low-fat diet can be one made of natural high-fiber, carb-rich foods like fruits, veggies, beans, and whole grains. However, soda, candy, and white bread/crackers/pasta are also low-fat foods, even though we should not be eating them every day. Cutting these processed foods out is likely why so many people are drawn to the Paleo diet. Refined and processed foods are not ideal for health—and especially not for weight loss. Eating

Paleo also means avoiding beans and whole grains. Cutting beans and whole grains out of the diet makes it very difficult to get enough fiber.

Kale, spinach, and other veggies do not come close to beans in terms of fiber.[19] In one cup, beans have five times more fiber than does cooked spinach.[19] Beans also have sixteen times more fiber than raw spinach has per cup.[19] So unless you eat sixteen cups of raw spinach, you cannot get as much fiber as someone eating one or two cups of beans each day.

Grams of Fiber Per Cup of Food

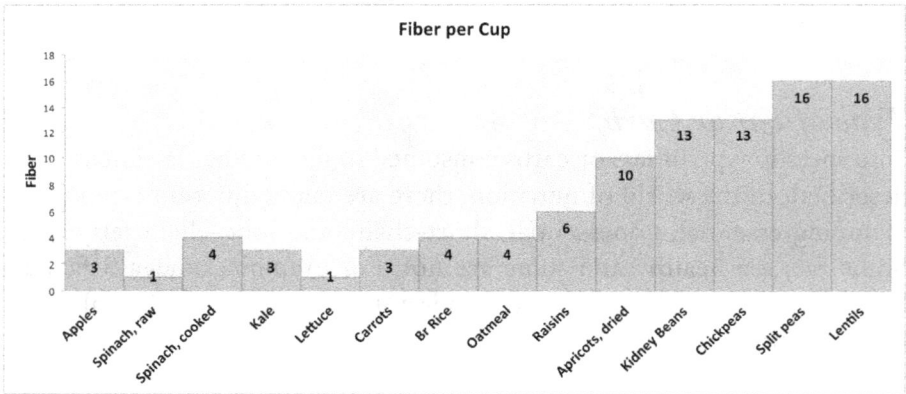

Data compiled by Jen Swallow from US Department of Agriculture, Agricultural Research Service. 2014. USDA National Nutrient Database for Standard Reference, Release 27. Nutrient Data Laboratory home page, http://www.ars.usda.gov/nutrientdata.

A low-fat diet filled with fruit, whole grains, beans, veggies, nuts, and seeds would inevitably have more fiber and less fat than any low-carb diet, even if it is compared with the Paleo diet. Future research should specify whether an experimental diet is low fat based on whole foods or low fat based on mostly processed foods. Whole foods are low in sugar and high in fiber compared with highly processed foods. They also tend to have more vitamins and minerals, such as vitamin C and potassium. When people eat whole foods, especially plant foods, they tend to eat fewer calories.

You're Not a Vulcan

Vulcans consistently use logic to make daily life choices. If you are familiar with *Star Trek*, you know how Vulcans have the ability to control their emotions. Humans, on the other hand, are easily overrun with emotions and desires. Think of friends or family members who have spent hard-earned money on a new smartphone, flat-screen TV, an expensive car, or jewelry that they cannot afford.

The excitement of something that looks good, tastes good, or feels good often takes over when we make decisions. This is why we often choose donuts over fruit and cheeseburgers over salads. Participants in research studies make mistakes even when they know the rules they are supposed to follow and which foods they are supposed to eat.

When an investigator calls participants to record what they ate, it's entirely plausible for them to forget or even lie. Can you remember what you ate yesterday or three days ago? What about a week ago? Keeping track of how much fat or what kind would be very difficult.

Measuring compliance to a diet is problematic because of human error and an unpredictable environment. There will always be some confounding factors despite how much researchers try to control for habits, age, health, and genetics of different people. Some subjects are more physically active than are others, and may therefore lose more weight, though they don't consider their activities to be real workouts. This is why it's important to review as many studies as possible to get a better idea of the big picture, which is how diet affects weight and overall health.

Short-Term Weight Loss

Diet studies are relatively short-term, lasting between six months and one year. Dieters aiming to lose weight are not imagining, "I will lose weight this year and then gain it all back next year." Who wants to work hard at reaching their skinny goal for a few months and then get fat again? This is exactly what happens, however, with most fad diets over time.

When four popular diets—Atkins, South Beach, Zone, and Weight Watchers—were compared by research scientists in Canada over a two-year period, all of them resulted in some weight loss.[21] Atkins had a larger range of weight loss, up to 10 lb in a year, while Weight Watchers was more *consistently* effective for weight loss.[21] They both also resulted in a partial regain of lost weight.[21]

Low Fat Can Work!

Plant-based diets commonly contain less fat than meat-centered diets. Vegans typically eat 5% of total calories as saturated fat, which is half of what Americans consume. They also eat less total fat and much more fiber when compared with Americans who eat a more traditional American diet.[1] Eating a lot of saturated fat, commonly found in meat, cheese, and butter, is associated with more body fat. In other words, eating high levels of fat can actually make people fat.[20] This kind of relationship does not happen for people who are cutting calories and purposely dieting. We are not talking about starving people in India here; we are talking about lazy, indulgent Americans.

If a starving underweight man eats a piece of fried sausage or even a stick of butter, he will still be skinny even if his diet is 100% saturated fat. The saturated fat dilemma is for those who eat food regularly and don't count calories. Short-term diets with calorie restrictions can work with any kind of mix of fat versus carbs or protein, which is why Paleo gurus can claim they have the solution to obesity.

Any trend or fad—such as fasting, juicing, meal replacements, low-carb diets, or surgery—can work for temporary weight loss. In reality, there is only so much bacon or steak smothered in butter a man can take before his body starts to reflect it. This kind of eating is not an effective long-term strategy for weight loss. Cutting down on saturated fat, on the other hand, does work for long-term weight loss.

Vegans and vegetarians in the United States tend to eat less fat than do omnivores and reap some benefits since they weigh less on average.[1] A low-fat diet may work as long as the type of fat is mostly from plants and the diet is generally a healthy one.

Conclusion

Diet study results often contradict one another because of inconsistent definitions, poor tracking of types/amount of foods, and the lack of long-term studies. The terms "low fat" and "low carb" do not necessarily mean that a diet is healthy. This is why it's important to review the details of each study before making rash decisions based on sensational headlines. The details can make a world of difference when it comes to drawing conclusions from research results. Claiming that participants on a low-carb diet lost weight or lowered their cholesterol is a vague and unspecific assertion. If a study completely omits the details, then there is no way to put this information into practice.

No matter what claim is made for diet studies, it is crucial to find very specific answers to all of these questions:

- Did investigators use a control diet or comparison diet?
- How many participants completed the study?
- How many calories did participants eat?
- How did participants track calories?
- Did participants do any kind of physical activity or exercises during the study?
- What specific kinds of foods did participants eat (e.g., how many fruits/veggies/etc.)?
- What percentage of calories from carbs or fat did participants eat?
- How much fiber did participants eat?
- How long did the study last?

Plenty of different methods can work for short-term weight loss including drugs, surgery, and dozens of diets. Low-carb diets are no exception to this phenomenon. This kind of weight loss, however, does not usually work for longer than a year. Compliance with radical diets becomes increasingly difficult in long-term settings, regardless of whether the diet is extremely low in carbs, fat, or total calories. Some rules, such as cutting out all carbs or cooked food or oil, can make long-term compliance tough. Choose a diet that gets results, improves your overall health, and lasts a lifetime.

Notes

1. Rizzo NS et al., "Nutrient profiles of vegetarian and nonvegetarian dietary patterns." *J Acad Nutr Diet* ,113 (2005): 1610–19.
2. "The Paleo Diet Premise," Loren Cordain, The Paleo Diet, Accessed February 10, 2015, http://thepaleodiet.com/the-paleo-diet-premise.
3. Rhyu HS, Cho SY, "The effect of weight loss by ketogenic diet on the body composition, performance-related physical fitness factors and cytokines of Taekwondo athletes," *J Exerc Rehabil*, 10 (2014): 326–31.
4. Nickols-Richardson SM, et al., "Perceived hunger is lower and weight loss is greater in overweight premenopausal women consuming a low-carbohydrate/high-protein vs high-carbohydrate/low-fat diet," *J Am Diet Assoc*, 105 (2004): 1433–37.
5. Halyburton AK, et al., "Low- and high-carbohydrate weight-loss diets have similar effects on mood but not cognitive performance." *Am J Clin Nutr*, 86 (2007): 580–87.
6. Daly, M.E. et al., "Short-term effects of severe dietary carbohydrate-restriction advice in Type 2 diabetes—a randomized controlled trial," *Diabet Med*, 23 (2006): 15–20.
7. J. Tay et al., "Metabolic effects of weight loss on a very-low-carbohydrate diet compared with an isocaloric high-carbohydrate diet in abdominally obese subjects," *J Am Coll Cardiol*, 51 (2008): 59–67.
8. Summer SS, et al.,"Adiponectin changes in relation to the macronutrient composition of a weight-loss diet," *Obesity (Silver Spring)*, 19 (2011): 2198–204.
9. Mueller-Cunningham WM, Quintana R, and Kasim-Karakas SE, "An ad libitum, very low-fat diet results in weight loss and changes

in nutrient intakes in postmenopausal women," *J Am Diet Assoc*, 103 (2003): 1600–6.

10. Krebs NF et al., "Efficacy and safety of a high protein, low carbohydrate diet for weight loss in severely obese adolescents," *J Pediatr*, 157 (2010): 252–58.

11. Brinkworth GD et al., "Long-term effects of a very low-carbohydrate diet and a low-fat diet on mood and cognitive function," *Arch Intern Med*, 169 (2009): 1873–80.

12. Alhassan S et al., "Dietary adherence and weight loss success among overweight women: results from the A to Z weight loss study," *Int J Obes (Lond)*, 32 (2008): 985–91.

13. Dansinger ML, et al., "Comparison of the Atkins, Ornish, Weight Watchers, and Zone diets for weight loss and heart disease risk reduction: a randomized trial," *JAMA*, 293 (2005): 43–53.

14. Foster GD, et al., "Weight and metabolic outcomes after 2 years on a low-carbohydrate versus low-fat diet: a randomized trial," *Ann Intern Med*, 153 (2010): 147–57.

15. Shai I, et al., "Weight loss with a low-carbohydrate, Mediterranean, or low-fat diet," *N Engl J Med*, 359 (2008): 229–41.

16. "Weekend Warrior Omelette," Loren Cordain, The Paleo Diet, Accessed February 10, 2015, http://thepaleodiet.com/weekend-warrior-omelette/.

17. "Mackerel Tartare: A Paleo Recipe for Common Cold Prevention," Christopher James Clark, The Paleo Diet, Accessed February 10, 2015, http://thepaleodiet.com/mackerel-tartare-paleo-recipe-common-cold-prevention.

18. "Paleo-Friendly One-Pot Meals," Loren Cordain, The Paleo Diet, Accessed February 10, 2015, http://thepaleodiet.com/paleo-friendly-one-pot-meals.

19. Data compiled by Jen Swallow from US Department of Agriculture, Agricultural Research Service. 2014. USDA National Nutrient Database for Standard Reference, Release 27. Nutrient Data Laboratory home page, Accessed February 14, 2015, http://www.ars.usda.gov/nutrientdata.

20. Varela-Moreiras G, "Controlling obesity: what should be changed?" *Int J Vitam Nutr Res*, 76 (2006): 262–68.
21. Atallah R, Filion KB, and Wakil SM, "Long term effect of 4 popular diets on weight loss and cardiovascular risk factors: a systemic review of randomized clinical trials," *Circ Cardiovasc Qual Outcomes*, 7 (2014): 815–27.

CHAPTER 4

What about Paleo?

A few studies have examined the effect of the Paleo diet on weight loss. Subjects eating the Paleo diet lost weight in short-term studies that utilized a very low-calorie intake.[1-4] In a real-world setting, food amount is not restricted and no one counts calories. In the Paleo diet, 55% of total calories come from meat,[5] but otherwise, dieters can eat as much Paleo-approved food as desired. This is how participants ate during a recent Paleo diet study, and despite losing 7 lb in two-and-a-half months, their bad (LDL) cholesterol and total cholesterol increased while good (HDL) cholesterol decreased.[6]

Summary of Paleo Diet Studies

Year	Author	Subjects	Length	Diet	Control	Results
2014	Boers et al[1]	32	2 wk	Paleo	Dutch Diet	Paleo= -3 lb, Dutch diet= -1 lb (both used 2000 calorie goal)
2008	Osterdahl et al[2]	14	1 mo	Paleo	None	Paleo= -5 lb (total calorie= 1584 cal, 24% protein, 36% fat, 40% carbs)
2007	Jonsson et al[3]	29	1.5 mo	Paleo	Mediterranean Diet	Paleo= -11 lb (1344 calories), Mediterranean= -9 lb.
2010	Jonsson et al[4]	29	3 mo	Paleo	Mediterranean Diet	Paleo group lost 5.6 cm in waist (1388 calories)
2014	Smith et al[5]	44	2.5 mo	Paleo	No control	Paleo= -7 lb, 3.6 % body fat

Paleo Diet Studies

Looking at weight loss over a six-month period is not very helpful to people who want their weight loss to be permanent over a period of years or decades. Any dietary method of weight loss, regardless of carb or fat content, can work for a few months as long as you stick to it. When calories consumed are lower than those burned, any diet can provide results. But will these results stand the test of time?

Paleo versus Vegan

A healthy plant-based diet, when done with 100% compliance, can be a very effective long-term cure for obesity. Unfortunately, subjects are not always compliant with their diets even during research studies. When the vegan diet is put to the test in a clinical setting, it can have varying results. In one study, a vegan group lost 16 lb in three months, in another they lost 17 lb in six months, and in yet another they lost only 10 lb in eighteen months.[6–11]

As with any diet, vegetarian or vegan diets work best when dieters independently commit to change rather than have scientists tell them to change for research purposes. People who seek weight-loss counseling and switch to a mostly vegan, plant-based diet can lose 50 lb in two years.[12] These contrasting results show that calories from fat—whether it is 10%, 20%, or 40% of total calories—does not matter as much as total calorie intake or physical activity when it comes to weight loss.

Plant-Based Diets and Weight Loss

Year	Author	Subjects	Length	Diet	Control	Results
1999	Nicholson et al[6]	11	3 mo	10% fat Vegan	30% low fat diet	Vegan group lost 16 lb, low fat diet lost 8 lb
2013	Mishra et al[7]	215	4.5 mo	10% fat Vegan	Control	Vegan group lost 9 lb, controls lost 0 lb
2009	Barnard et al[8]	99	1.5 yr	10% fat vegan	ADA diet	Vegan group lost 10 lb, ADA group lost 7 lb
2007	Jenkins et al[9]	23	6 mo	Low carb vegan	Vegetarian diet	Vegan group lost 15 lb, Vegetarian group lost 13 lb.
2007	Burke et al[10]	176	1.5 yr	Low fat vegetarian	25% low fat diet	Both groups lost 17 lb with calorie restriction (1200-1500w, 1500-1800m calories)
2015	Turner-McGrievy et al[11]	63	6 mo	10% fat vegan	Omni/Veg or pesco veg	Vegan group lost 17 lb, omnivore group lost 7 lb

Reducing Meat Protein for Weight Loss

High-protein diets based around meat may work in the short-term while the motivation to cut calories is strong. A few months into dieting, however, most people tend not to stick to the high-protein, low-carb rules. Even if they did, the extra calories that come along with protein tend to add up. Meat is not made of pure protein; it also has fat, which is dense in calories. Protein from plants, such as beans and whole grains, does not contain significant amounts of fat. Plants have some carbs, which are lower per gram when compared with fat. This is one reason why a plant-based diet beats out regular omnivorous diets for weight loss. When it comes to long-term protection from obesity, low-carb diets simply do not have the track record that plant-based diets have.[12-14]

Staying thin year after year is more difficult for those on a high-fat/protein diet,[13, 14] which is what low-carb meals tend to be. Generally, the more plant foods and fewer animal foods people eat, the slimmer they are.[15-20] Junk-food carbs like soda and candy (which vegetarians and vegans can still eat) are not helpful for weight loss, of course, but most plant foods that are not junk foods do work well.

While this trend in research does not prove that vegans are always slimmer than meat eaters, it does suggest that staying thin is more likely to happen on a vegetarian or vegan diet compared with a meat-eating diet.[21-29] People who avoid animal products—vegans—are consistently slimmer than vegetarians and meat eaters. [21-29] This fact is evident when looking at major studies from Europe, the United States, and Canada.[21-29] (See the following table for a comparison of BMI between meat eaters and vegetarians/vegans. BMI is body mass index, which is a rough estimate of body fat using a ratio of weight to height.)

BMI of Meat Eaters versus Vegetarians and Vegans

Year	Country	Author	Subjects	Vegan	Vegetarian	Omnivore
2014	UK	Bradbury et al[21]	600 men	22 normal	23 normal	25 overweight
2013	US/Canada	Tonstad et al[22]	49,000 adults	24 normal	25 overweight	28 overweight
2010	Europe	Gilsing et al[23]	700 men	22 normal	23 normal	26 overweight
2009	US	Robinson et al[24]	1600 adults	23 normal	24 normal	25 overweight
2009	US	Tonstad et al[25]	60,000 adults	24 normal	26 overweight	29 overweight
2006	US	Rosell et al[26]	10,000 men	23 normal	24 normal	26 overweight
2006	US	Rosell et al[26]	10,000 women	23 normal	24 normal	25 overweight
2005	US	Newby et al[27]	55,459 adults	23 normal	23 normal	25 overweight
2003	UK	Spencer et al[28]	38,000 adults	22 normal	23 normal	26 overweight
1995	Canada	Janelle et al[29]	45 healthy mix	21 normal	21 normal	23 normal

Keeping the Weight Off

The studies discussed in this chapter have been small and relatively short-lived. Only a few have included more than two hundred people and lasted longer than a year. Even two hundred subjects comprise a small group when the whole US population is taken into consideration. Keep in mind that there are over 320 million Americans, so it's difficult to imagine how small clinical studies of two hundred or three hundred people can relate to hundreds of millions of adults.

Losing weight for a year or two before regaining it all is a waste of effort. Wouldn't it be great to see how people lose weight and keep it off for more than five years or even a decade? Actually, there is a group of research participants who fit these criteria well. The National Weight

Control Registry (NWCR) was created by Brown Medical School and the University of Colorado to track long-term weight-loss maintenance in ten thousand subjects.[13] The average NWCR participant has maintained a weight loss of 60 lb for five years.[13]

The majority of successful NWCR weight losers were eating a low-fat diet; many reported eating 24% of total calories as fat.[13–15] Those who regained some weight tended to report a decrease in physical activity and an increase in eating fat as the reason for the relapse.[14, 15] Though *some* NWCR participants lost weight with a low-carb diet, they represent only a fraction of successful registry participants.[13, 14]

The NWCR findings are consistent with survey results from the general US population. High-carbohydrate diets have long been linked to maintaining a healthy weight. The federal government gathers information about the US population through surveys about food choices and dietary intake to assess how diet affects health. USDA researchers analyzed the diets of 10,000 American adults who followed low-carb, high-carb, or a vegetarian diet.[16] They found that vegetarians and the high-carb group were the leanest.[16] The low-carb group had the most overweight and obese people.[16]

While eating more fat is not guaranteed to make people fat, it has a tendency to lead to long-term weight gain, especially in sedentary people.[14–18] Americans are not the only ones affected by this relationship between dietary fat and body fat. A British survey of over two thousand adults showed that those eating a high-fat diet (45% fat) were more likely to be overweight or obese compared with those eating a moderate-fat diet (35% or less).[17]

Notes

1. Boers I, et al., "Favourable effects of consuming a Paleolithic-type diet on characteristics of the metabolic syndrome: a randomized controlled pilot-study," *Lipids Health Dis*, 13 (2014): 160.

2. Osterdahl M, et al., "Effects of a short-term intervention with a Paleolithic diet in healthy volunteers," *Eur J Clin Nutr*, 62 (2008): 682–85.

3. Lindeberg S, et al., "A Paleolithic diet improves glucose tolerance more than a Mediterranean-like diet in individuals with ischaemic heart disease," *Diabetologia*, 50 (2007): 1795–807.

4. Jonsson T, et al., "A Paleolithic diet is more satiating per calorie than a Mediterranean-like diet in individuals with ischemic heart disease," *Nutr Metab*, 30 (2010): 85.

5. "The Paleo Diet Premise," Loren Cordain, The Paleo Diet, Accessed February 10, 2015, http://thepaleodiet.com/the-paleo-diet-premise.

6. Smith M, et al., "Unrestricted Paleolithic diet is associated with unfavorable changes to blood lipids in healthy subjects," *Intl J Exerc Sci*, 7 (2014): 128–139.

7. Nicholson AS, et al., "Toward improved management of NIDDM: A randomized, controlled, pilot intervention using a lowfat, vegetarian diet," *Prev Med*; 29 (1999): 87–91.

8. Mishra S, et al., "Nutrient intake in the GEICO multicenter trial: the effects of a multicomponent worksite intervention," *Eur J Clin Nutr*, 67 (2013): 1066–71.

9. Barnard ND, et al., "A low-fat vegan diet and a conventional diabetes diet in the treatment of type 2 diabetes: a randomized, controlled, 74-wk clinical trial," *Am J Clin Nutr*, 89 (2009): 1588S–1596S.

10. Jenkins DJ, et al., "Effect of a 6-month vegan low-carbohydrate ('Eco-Atkins') diet on cardiovascular risk factors and body weight in hyperlipidaemic adults: a randomized controlled trial," *BMJ*, 4 (2014): e003505.

11. Burke LE, et al., "Effects of a vegetarian diet and treatment preference on biochemical and dietary variables in overweight and obese adults: a randomized clinical trial," *Am J Clin Nutr*, 86 (2007): 588–96.

12. Turner-McGrievy GM, et al., "Comparative effectiveness of plant-based diets for weight loss: A randomized controlled trial of five different diets," *Nutrition*, 31 (2015): 350–58.

13. Sarter B, Campbell TC, and Fuhrman J, "Effect of a high nutrient density diet on long-term weight loss: a retrospective chart review," *Altern Ther Health Med*, 14 (2008): 48–53.

14. Thomas JG, et al., "Weight-loss maintenance for 10 years in the National Weight Control Registry," *Am J Prev Med*, 46 (2014): 17–23.

15. McGuire MT, et al., "What predicts weight regain in a group of successful weight losers?" *J Consult Clin Psychol*, 67 (1999): 177–85.

16. Shick SM, et al., "Persons successful at long-term weight loss and maintenance continue to consume a low-energy, low-fat diet," *J Am Diet Assoc*, 98 (1988): 408–13.

17. Kennedy ET, et al., "Popular diets correlation to health, nutrition, and obesity," *J Am Diet Assoc*, 101 (2001): 411–20.

18. Macdiarmid JI, Cade JE, and Blundell JE, "High and low fat consumers, their macronutrient intake and body mass index: further analysis of the National Diet and Nutrition Survey of British Adults," *Eur J Clin Nutr*, 50 (1996): 505–12.

19. Corella D et al., "A high intake of saturated fatty acids strengthens the association between the fat mass and obesity-associated gene and BMI," *J Nutr*, 14 (2011): 2219–25.

20. Timpson NJ, et al., "The fat mass- and obesity-associated locus and dietary intake in children," *Am J Clin Nutr*, 88 (2008): 971–78.

21. Bradbury KE, Crowe FL, Appleby PN, Schmidt JA, Travis RC, Key TJ. "Serum concentrations of cholesterol, apolipoprotein A-1 and apolipoprotein B in a total of 1694 meat-eaters, fish-eaters, vegetarians and vegans." *Eur J Clin Nutr* 2014; 68 (2): 178-83.

22. Tonstad SI, Stewart K, Oda K, Batech M, Herring RP, Fraser GE. "Vegetarian diets and incidence of diabetes in the Adventist Health Study-2." *Nutr Metab Cardiovasc* 2013; 23 (4): 292-9.

23. Gilsing AMJ, Crowe FL, Lloyd-Wright Z, Sanders TAB, Appleby PN, Allen NE, Key TJ. "Serum concentrations of vitamin B12 and folate in British male omnivores, vegetarians and vegans: a result from a cross-sectional analysis of the EPIC-Oxford cohort study." *Eur J Clin Nutr* 2010; 64 (9): 933-939.

24. Robinson-O'Brien R, Perry CL, Wall MM, Story M, Neumark-Sztainer D. "Adolescent and young adults vegetarianism: better

dietary intake and weight outcomes but increased risk of disordered eating behaviors." *J Am Diet Assoc* 2009; 109 (4): 648-655.

25. Tonstad S, Butler T, Yan R, Fraser GE. "Types of vegetarian diet, body weight, and prevalence of type 2 diabetes." *Diabetes Care* 2009; 32 (5): 791-6.

26. Rosell M, Appleby P, Spencer E, Key T. "Weight gain over 5 years in 21,966 meat-eating, fish-eating, vegetarian, and vegan men and women in EPIC-Oxford." *Int J Obes* 2006; 30: 1389-1396.

27. Newby PK, Tucker KL, Wolk A. "Risk of overweight and obesity among semivegetarian, lactovegetarian, and vegan women." Am J Clin Nutr 2005;81(6):1267-74.

28. Spencer EA Int, Appleby PN, Davey GK, Key TJ. "Diet and body mass index in 38000 EPIC-Oxford meat-eaters, fish-eaters, vegetarians and vegans." *Int J Obes Relat Metab Disord* 2003; 27 (6): 728-34.

29. Janelle KC, Barr SI. "Nutrient intakes and eating behavior scores of vegetarian and nonvegetarian women." *J Am Diet Assoc* 1995; 95 (2): 180-6.

CHAPTER 5

You're Not a Masai Man

You are not part of the Masai tribe living in Africa, or are you? If you are, then you might eat as much meat and dairy as you can without consequence. The low-carb diet is truly put into practice in this culture. Low-carb enthusiasts mention the Masai tribal community of East Africa as an example of how eating saturated fat and cholesterol is harmless.

The traditional Masai diet is high in fat with 66% of calories from fat and over 600 mg of cholesterol per day because the diet is composed of mostly milk and meat.[1] This is double the amount Americans eat of both fat and cholesterol.[2] Yet when the average cholesterol level among Masai of various ages was analyzed in the early 1970s, it was a mere 135 mg/dL compared with the current 200 mg/dL average in America.[1, 3]

If saturated fat raises cholesterol, how is this Masai phenomenon possible?

The answer is genetics. The Masai have special genes that allow them to make less cholesterol while compensating for the high intake.[1] This compensation does not occur as efficiently with pregnant Masai women as their cholesterol levels are much higher.[1] When other African tribes eating the same diet are compared with the Masai, such as the Samburu and Rendille of northern Kenya, they have higher cholesterol levels.[1]

Americans clearly don't have these special genes. We eat less than half the cholesterol and saturated fat that the Masai eat but still have much higher blood cholesterol levels and a higher prevalence of heart disease.[1-3] Adult men in the United States eat about 300 mg of cholesterol and 34% fat on average.[2]

You're Not an Eskimo

You also are probably not an Eskimo, though this is more likely than the caveman scenario. The Alaskan or Greenland Eskimos, also known as Inuit, are another example of a large population eating a low-carb diet. Fish, seals, and seafood make up a large portion of the Inuit diet.[4]

Fish is a popular source of an essential fat that is known as omega-3 fat. The daily Inuit diet has 3–14 g of omega-3 fat in contrast to 0.2 g in the American diet.[4,5] This means the Inuit eat at least ten times more omega-3 fat when compared with Americans.[4,5] Does this low-carb Inuit diet truly protect the heart, and does it work for weight loss? Is the traditional Inuit diet anything like the modern Paleo diet?

Butter, bacon, grass-fed beef, and eggs were not a major part of the original Inuit diet as they are in the modern Paleo diet.[4] The Inuit eat less saturated fat (9%) than non-Inuit Americans (12%).[4] This is vastly different from the Paleo diet, which is high in saturated fat from pork, beef, and lamb.

Looking at data from the past forty years, Alaskan and Canadian Inuit did not have lower rates of heart disease when compared with modern-day Americans.[5,6] Autopsies on Alaskan natives in the late 1980s show that while they had heart disease, it seemed to progress slower than in nonnatives.[7] This phenomenon can be explained partially by the difference in diet, omega-3 intake, and genetics.

Inuit genes and their omega-3 intake were slightly protective. As the traditional Inuit diet was influenced by Western foods, blood cholesterol worsened in this population.[8] Genetically mixed Inuit have lower HDL (good) cholesterol when compared with genetically pure Inuit.[8] Since HDL offers some protection as long as total cholesterol is not through the roof, we can conclude that there is some level of genetic protection offered by being from a pure Inuit family. Today, Alaskan Inuit are affected by heart disease much like regular Americans despite a seafood-rich diet.[6, 9–11]

In 2008, researchers at the Norton Sound Health Corporation in Alaska tested over 1,000 Alaskan Eskimos for heart disease.[6] They used food-frequency questionnaires for estimating dietary intake and ultrasound technology to detect plaque buildup in the carotid arteries.[6] Norton researchers found that omega-3 fat intake did not affect the amount of plaque found in arteries, but saturated fat intake was linked to plaque buildup.[6] In other words, Eskimos who ate more saturated fat had more clogged arteries, and omega-3 intake did not reduce the amount of clogged arteries.[6]

Now we know that the Inuit had heart disease despite their high intake of omega-3. But how did this low-carb diet affect obesity? Are traditional Inuit slimmer than regular Americans? Inuit eating the traditional diet are *not* thin. Despite a low-carb, high-protein diet, the Inuit are as fat as Americans with the same rate of cancer, and they do not live longer than the average American.[12–14] Some of the cancer prevalence is due to smoking, which is common in this population. This is one reason why the life expectancy of Canadian Inuit is ten years lower (sixty-six years) than non-Inuit Canadians (seventy-six years).[13] However, even after controlling for smoking, a traditional Inuit diet is actually linked to increased inflammation.[15]

Which Foods Raise Cholesterol?

Using the Masai tribe and Inuit as examples, the Paleo diet has given bacon, grass-fed beef, and eggs renewed popularity. After all, if the Masai and

Inuit can eat tons of fat and cholesterol without consequences, why can't we? How does a high-fat diet affect us in the long-term and in the absence of weight loss? Of course *during* weight loss, blood pressure, cholesterol, and blood sugars decrease, but what happens *after*?

There are many factors that can affect cholesterol, including being overweight and obesity. No matter what you eat, if you are obese, you are at an increased risk of heart disease and total mortality. Diet is a major factor, along with weight, that affects cholesterol. Some humans have unique genes that make them more sensitive or less sensitive to foods that raise cholesterol. When it comes to having the genes that make them less sensitive, the Masai and Inuit are rare exceptions to a general rule. According to new research, eating fat, particularly saturated fat, raises cholesterol.[16-25]

The effect of eating saturated fat on blood cholesterol is supported by overwhelming new and long-standing research from around the world.[16-25] If eating this way only affected Americans, then we could conclude that our genes make us particularly sensitive to this kind of diet. The fact is that saturated fat has the same kind of effect on cholesterol across a wide spectrum of different genes.[16-25]

British, Austrian, Finnish, and Japanese people experience a rise in cholesterol with a rise in saturated fat intake.[16-25] Take a look at the following chart with several current and old studies from different countries that came to the same conclusion about how eating saturated fat is linked to blood cholesterol.

Dietary Fat and Blood Cholesterol

Year	Location	Authors	Subject #	Findings
2015	Australia	Blekkenhorst et al[16]	1469	Saturated fat intake was linked to total & LDL cholesterol; >31g/day tripled the mortality risk vs 5g sat fat intake
2011	UK	Hooper et al[17]	65,000	Low cholesterol level tied to low saturated fat intake
2013	Austria	Schwingshackl et al[18]	8,000	Low cholesterol level tied to low saturated fat intake
1996	Finland	Schwab et al[19]	12	Palmitic acid intake raised cholesterol
1996	Netherlands	Temme et al[20]	32	Saturated fat raised cholesterol
2009	Denmark	Jakobsen et al[21]	340,000	Replacing saturated with polyunsaturated fat lowered heart disease risk
2014	USA	Farvid et al[22]	310,000	Replacing saturated with polyunsaturated fat lowered risk of heart disease death by 13%
2010	UK	Donin et al[23]	2,000	Low cholesterol is due to low saturated fat intake
2005	Japan	Adachi et al[24]	2,000	Fat intake, especially saturated fat, increased from 5 to 20%, mean cholesterol increased from 152 to 194 mg/dL in adults
1982	Japan	Ueshima et al[25]	2,000	Adults eating 14% fat had a lower mean cholesterol (165 mg/dL) than those eating 23% fat (202 mg/dL cholesterol)
2001	New Zealand	Hodson et al[26]	70	Replacing saturated with unsaturated fat lowers cholesterol

Cholesterol versus Mortality

Can we predict disease and mortality by looking at cholesterol levels? Yes, in a way we can evaluate whether someone is in danger of experiencing a heart attack by looking at that person's blood cholesterol levels.[27-38] Since heart disease is the most common killer of Americans, this is a fundamental concept for health.[39] Cholesterol is not the only test that helps estimate risk, but it remains an important one.[27-38] There are many blood tests that can help reveal the risk of heart disease, but the most common group of tests is in the lipid panel, which includes total, LDL, and HDL cholesterol counts along with triglycerides.

An overwhelming amount of new and old research from around the world has shown a correlation between high cholesterol and heart disease.[27-37] In other words, people from nearly all genetic backgrounds are affected by cholesterol levels.[27-37] Genes can influence health, but diet is usually a stronger factor in the prevalence of heart disease. In the end, eating more saturated fat means having high blood cholesterol for most people,[16-26] and high cholesterol is associated with death from heart disease.[27-38] This relationship is stronger in adults under the age of fifty-five.[39]

Here are multiple studies that indicate total cholesterol, LDL cholesterol, and total-to-HDL cholesterol ratios are effective for predicting heart attacks or death from heart disease.

Cholesterol Level and Heart Attacks

Year	Location	Authors	Subject #	Findings
2009	Japan	Okamura et al[27]	4,600	High LDL cholesterol associated with heart attacks
2013	Iran	Tohidi et al [28]	2,600	Total and LDL cholesterol predicted heart attacks
2010	Iran	Tohidi et al[29]	6,000	Total , LDL cholesterol, and triglycerides predicted heart attacks
2014	Japan	Takeuchi et al[30]	26,000	LDL cholesterol was associated with heart disease
2000	USA	Ridker et al[31]	28,000	Hs-CRP and total cholesterol to HDL ratio predicted heart attacks
2014	China	Ding et al[32]	1,900	LDL cholesterol was linked to all-cause mortality
2010	Finland	Taskinen et al[33]	9,700	Total to HDL cholesterol ratio predicted heart attacks in diabetics
2014	UK	Batty et al[34]	15,000	Total cholesterol linked to heart disease in men under 30 years
2013	Norway	Holme et al[35]	14,000	Total cholesterol linked to heart disease mortality
2010	China	Li et al[36]	5,000	Total cholesterol predicted heart attacks
2015	USA	Pikula et al[37]	6,000	Total, LDL, and total to HDL ratio predicted heart attacks
2015	Denmark	Varbo et al[38]	90,000	LDL cholesterol tied to heart attacks

A total-to-HDL cholesterol ratio above 5 is likely to predict a heart attack.[36] For example, my ratio is very close to 2 because my HDL is 51 and my total is 110; therefore, I am not at high risk for heart disease. Although this ratio is a better biomarker for heart disease, the other tests are also important.[36] Total cholesterol and LDL cholesterol are particularly significant for those who already have high blood pressure or another risk factor for heart disease.[35]

Does Cholesterol Size or Number Matter?

Some Paleo advocates claim that routine cholesterol blood tests are virtually useless, especially total cholesterol.[41] They believe that bad cholesterol—LDL—is unimportant because as long as good cholesterol—HDL—is high it will protect people from a heart attack. They also think that the size of LDL particles is more important than the number.[40] But as we saw in the table above, all of the numbers matter, so *quantity* is still important when it comes to cholesterol level.

Both LDL cholesterol size and number are good indicators of heart disease.[42, 43] LDL size, however, may be a *stronger* predictor of heart attacks.[41–45] Canadian researchers found that men with small LDL particles have double the risk of heart disease than those with larger LDL particles.[44] Though large particles are not as dangerous as small LDL, they are both bad because neither one is completely innocuous. But LDL cholesterol level is still an independent predictor, even more so than other lipids, such as triglycerides.[42]

This relationship between cholesterol and mortality exists for young adults and middle-aged adults under fifty-five, but it does not work quite the same way for the elderly.[46] For those above the age of sixty-five, for example, the relationship between high cholesterol and mortality changes.[46] Seniors tend to have higher mortality with low-cholesterol levels.[46–47] Low cholesterol, especially low HDL cholesterol, is an indicator of frailty and risk for infection in the elderly.[48–49] It is best to keep a moderate level of cholesterol during this stage of life because mortality is linked with very high or very low levels.[50]

As people age, they tend to be less physically active, lose their appetites, and eat less, which exacerbates their frailty. This is the opposite of health problems faced by young and middle-aged adults in the United States who struggle with weight gain. Loss of appetite in the elderly leads to weight loss, which results in low blood pressure, anemia, low protein status, and low cholesterol. These issues are all too familiar to me working around geriatric patients. I see patients with anemia and low cholesterol quite often.

At the last stage of life, it is too late to be worrying about cholesterol levels. Heart disease starts during childhood,[51, 52] so by the time a person has reached sixty, the disease would already have had plenty of time to progress. Once the arteries are clogged, in other words, testing cholesterol level is less useful. The best time to take charge of health and make lifestyle changes is between youth and middle age. During that time, a combination of eating more produce, not smoking, and eating less cholesterol and saturated fat can make more of an impact than drug use alone.[53]

A population in Finland illustrates this point well. Adults there experienced a 20% decrease in total cholesterol levels, mostly due to a decline in saturated fat and cholesterol intake.[53, 54] Cholesterol levels dropped by an average of 38 mg/dL over the span of a few decades.[53, 54] The change in dietary fat and cholesterol accounted for most of that drop.[53, 54] The rest of the change was likely due to an increase in fruit and vegetable consumption, an increase in medication use, and a decrease in smoking.[53] Heart disease mortality subsequently decreased by over 50% along with the decline in dietary fat and cholesterol.[54]

Notes

1. Taylor CB, Ho KJ. "Studies on the Masai." *Am J Clin Nutr* 1971: 1291-93.
2. "What We Eat in America 2011-2012", USDA Food Surveys, Accessed September 5, 2015, http://ars.usda.gov/Services/docs. htm?docid=13793.
3. Carroll MD, Lacher DA, Sorlie PD, Cleeman JI, Gordon DJ, Wolz M, et al. "Trends in serum lipids and lipoproteins of adults, 1960-2002." *JAMA* 2005; 294 (14): 1773-81.
4. Feskens EJ, Kromhout D. "Epidemiologic studies on Eskimos and fish intake." *Ann N Y Acad Sci* 1993; 683: 9-15.

5. Fodor JG, Helis E, Yazdekhasti N, Vohnout B. "Fishing for the origins of the "Eskimos and heart disease" story: facts or wishful thinking? *Can J Cardiol* 2014; 30 (8): 864-8.

6. Ebbesson SO, Roman MJ, Devereux RB, Kaufman D, Fabsitz RR, Maccluer JW, et al. "Consumption of omega-3 fatty acids is not associated with a reduction in carotid atherosclerosis: the Genetics of Coronary Artery Disease in Alaska Natives study." *Atherosclerosis* 2008; 199 (2): 346-53.

7. McLaughlin J, Middaugh J, Boudreau D, Malcom G, Parry S, Tracy R, Newman W. "Adipose tissue triglyceride fatty acids and atherosclerosis in Alaska Natives and non-Natives." *Atherosclerosis* 2005; 181 (2): 353-62.

8. Bierregaard P, Jorgensen ME, Borch-Johnsen K. "Serum lipids of Greenland Inuit in relation to Inuit genetic heritage, westernization and migration." *Atherosclerosis* 2004; 174 (2): 391-8.

9. Redwood DG, Lanier AP, Johnston JM, Asay ED, Slattery ML. "Chronic disease risk factors among Alaska Native and American Indian people, Alaska, 2004-2006." *Prev Chronic Dis* 2010; 7 (4): A85.

10. Ebbesson SO, Risica PM, Ebbesson LO, Kennish JM. "Eskimos have CHD despite high consumption of omega-3 fatty acids: the Alaska Siberia project." *Int J Circumpolar Health* 2005; 64 (4): 387-95.

11. Bjerregaard P, Young TK, Hegele RA. "Low incidence of cardiovascular disease among the Inuit—what is the evidence?" *Atherosclerosis* 2003; 166 (2): 351-7.

12. Young TK. "Obesity, central fat patterning, and their metabolic correlates among the Inuit of the central Canadian Arctic." *Hum Biol* 1996; 68 (2): 245-63.

13. Wilkins R, Uppal S, Fines P, Senecal S, Guimond E, Dion R. "Life expectancy in the Inuit-inhabited areas of Canada, 1989 to 2003." *Health Rep* 2008; 19 (1): 7-19.

14. Lanier AP, Blot WJ, Bender TR, Fraumeni JF. "Cancer in Alaskan Indians, Eskimos, and Aleuts." *J Natl Cancer Inst* 1980; 65 (5): 1157-9

15. Schaebel LH, Vestergaard H, Laurberg P, Rathcke CN, Andersen S. "Intake of traditional Inuit diet vary in parallel with inflammation as estimated from YKL-40 and hsCRP in Inuit and non-Inuit in Greenland." *Atherosclerosis* 2013; 228 (2): 496-501.
16. Blekkenhorst LC, Prince RL, Hodgson JM, Lim WH, Zhu K, Devine A, et al. "Dietary saturated fat intake and atherosclerotic vascular disease mortality in elderly women: a prospective cohort study." *Am Soc Nutr* 2015. Doi:10.3945/ ajcn.114.102392.
17. Hooper L, Summerbell CD, Thompson R, Sills D, Roberts FG, Moore H, et al. "Reduced or modified dietary fat for preventing cardiovascular disease." *Cochrane Database Syst Rev* 2011; (7): CD002137.
18. Schwingshackl L, Hoffman G. "Comparison of effects of long-term low-fat diets on blood lipid levels in overweight or obese patients: a systemic review and meta-analysis." *J Acad Nutr Diet* 2013; 113 (12): 1640-61.
19. Schwab US, Maliranta HM, Sarkkinen ES, Savolainen MJ, Kesaniemi YA, Uusitupa MI. "Different effects of palmitic and stearic-enriched diets on serum lipids and lipoproteins and plasma cholesteryl ester transfer protein activity in healthy young women." *Metabolism* 1996; 45 (2): 143-9.
20. Temme EH, Mensink RP, Hornstra G. "Comparison of the effects of diets enriched in lauric, palmitic, or oleic acids on serum lipids and lipoproteins in healthy women and men." *Am J Clin Nutr* 1996; 63 (6): 897-903.
21. Jakobsen MU, O'Reilly EJ, Heitmann BL, Pereira MA, Balter K, Fraser GE, et al. "Major types of dietary fat and risk of coronary heart disease: a pooled analysis of 11 cohort studies." *Am J Clin Nutr* 2009; 89 (5): 1425-32.
22. Farvid MS, Ding M, Pan A, Sun Q, Chiuve SE, Steffen LM, et al. "Dietary linoleic acid and risk of coronary heart disease: a systematic review and meta-analysis of prospective cohort studies." *Circulation* 2014 [Epub ahead of print]
23. Donin AS, Nightingale CM, Owen CG, Rudnicka AR, McNamara MC, Prynne CJ, et al. "Ethnic differences in blood lipids and dietary intake between UK children of black African, black Caribbean,

South Asian, and white European origin: the Child Heart and Health Study in England (CHASE)." *Am J Clin Nutr* 2010; 92 (4): 776-83.

24. Adachi H, Hino A. "Trends in nutritional intake and serum cholesterol levels over 40 years in Tanushimaru, Japanese men." *J Epidemiol* 2005; 15 (3): 85-9.

25. Ueshima H, Lida M, Shimamoto T, Konishi M, Tanigaki M, Doi M, et al. "Dietary intake and serum total cholesterol level: their relationship to different lifestyles in several Japanese populations." *Circulation* 1982;66(3):519-26.

26. Hodson L, Skeaff CM, Chisholm WA. "The effect of replacing dietary saturated fat with polyunsaturated or monounsaturated fat on plasma lipids in free-living young adults." *Eur J Clin Nutr* 2001; 55 (10): 908-15.

27. Okamura T, Kokubo Y, Watanabe M, Higashiyama A, Miyamoto Y, Yoshimasa Y, et al. "Low-density lipoprotein cholesterol and non-high-density lipoprotein cholesterol and the incidence of cardiovascular disease in an urban Japanese cohort study: The Suita study." *Atherosclerosis* 2009; 203 (2): 587-92.

28. Tohidi M, Mohebi R, Cheraghi L, Haisheikholeslami F, Aref S, Nouri S, et al. "Lipid profile components and incident cerebrovascular events versus coronary heart disease: the result of 9 years of follow-up in Tehran Lipid and Glucose Study." *Clin Biochem* 2013; 46 (9): 716-21.

29. Tohidi M, Hatami M, Hadaegh F, Safarkhani M, Harati H, Azizi F. "Lipid measures for prediction of incident cardiovascular disease in diabetic and non-diabetic adults: results of the 8.6 years follow-up of a population based cohort study." *Lipids Health Dis* 2010; 9: 6.

30. Takeuchi T, Nemoto K, Takahashi O, Urayama KY, Deshpande GA, Izumo H. "Comparison of cardiovascular disease risk associated with 3 lipid measures in Japanese adults." *J Clin Lipidol* 2014.8 (5) : 501-9.

31. Ridker PM, Hennekens CH, Buring JE, Rifai N. "C-reactive protein and other markers of inflammation in the prediction of cardiovascular disease in women." *N Engl J Med* 2000; 342 (12): 836-43.

32. Ding D, Li X, Qiu J, Li R, Zhang Y, Su D, et al. "Serum lipids, apolipoproteins, and mortality among coronary artery disease patients." *Biomed Res Int* 2014. [Epub ahead of print.]

33. Taskinen MR, Barter PJ, Ehnholm C, Sullivan DR, Mann K, Simes J, et al. "Ability of traditional lipid ratios and apolipoprotein ratios to predict cardiovascular risk in people with type 2 diabetes." *Diabetologia* 2010; 53 (9): 1846-55.

34. Batty GD, Shipley M, Davey Smith G, Kivimaki M. "Long term risk factors for coronary heart disease and stroke: influence of duration of follow-up over four decades of mortality surveillance." *Eur J Prev Cardiol* 2014. [Epub ahead of print.]

35. Holme I, Tonstad S. "Association of coronary heart disease mortality with risk factors according to length of follow-up and serum cholesterol level in men: the Oslo Study cohort." *Eur J Prev Cardiol* 2013; 20 (1): 168-75.

36. Li JX, Cao J, Chen SF, Yu DH, Duan XF, Wu XG, Gu DF. "The effect of total cholesterol on myocardial infarction in Chinese male hypertension population." *Biomed Environ Sci* 2010; 23 (1): 37-41.

37. Pikula A, Beiser AS, Wang J, Himali JJ, Kelly-Hayes M, Kase CS, et al. "Lipid and lipoprotein measurements and the risk of ischemic vascular events: Framingham Study." *Neurology* 2015; 84 (5): 472-9.

38. Varbo A, Freiberg JJ, Nordestgaard BG. "Extreme nonfasting remnant cholesterol vs extreme LDL cholesterol as contributors to cardiovascular disease and all-cause mortality in 90,000 individuals from the general population." *Clin Chem* 2015; 61 (3): 533-43.

39. "Leading Causes of Death", Centers for Disease Control and Prevention, Accessed March 6, 2015, http://www.cdc.gov/nchs/fastats/leading-causes-of-death.htm.

40. Frost PH, Verter J, Miller D. "Serum lipids and lipoproteins after myocardial infarction: association with cardiovascular mortality and experience in the Aspirin Myocardial Infarction Study." *Am Heart J* 1987; 113 (6): 1356-64.

41. "The Diet-Heart Myth: Why Everyone Should Know Their LDL Particle Number", Chris Kresser, Accessed March 9, 2015,

42. http://chriskresser.com/the-diet-heart-myth-why-everyone-should-know-their-ldl-particle-number/.

43. Shoji T, Hatsuda S, Tsuchikura S, Shinohara K, Kimoto E, Koyama H, et al. "Small dense low-density lipoprotein cholesterol concentration and carotid atherosclerosis." *Atherosclerosis* 2009; 202 (2): 582-8.

44. Berneis K, Jeanneret C, Muser J Felix B, Miserez AR. "Low-density lipoprotein size and subclasses are markers of clinically apparent and non-apparent atherosclerosis in type 2 diabetes." *Metabolism* 2005; 54 (2): 227-34.

45. Lamarche B, St-Pierre AC, Ruel IL, Cantin B, Dagenais GR, Despres JP. "A prospective, population-based study of low density lipoprotein particle size as a risk factor for ischemic heart disease in men." *Can J Cardiol* 2001; 17 (8): 859-65.

46. Aoki T, Yagi H, Sumino H, Tsunekawa K, Araki O, Kimura T, et al. "Relationship between carotid artery intima-media thickness and small dense low-density lipoprotein cholesterol concentrations measured by homogenous assay in Japanese subjects." *Clin Chim Acta* 2015; 442: 110-4.

47. Onder G, Landi F, Volpato S, Fellin R, Carbonin P, Gambassi G, etal. "Serum cholesterol levels and in-hospital mortality in the elderly." *Am J Med* 2003; 115 (4): 265-271.

48. Lv YB, Yin ZX, Chei CL, Qian HZ, Kraus VB, Zhang J, et al. "Low-density lipoprotein cholesterol was inversely associated with 3-year all-cause mortality among Chinese oldest old: Data from the Chinese Longitudinal Healthy Longevity Survey." 2015; 239 (1): 137-42.

49. Schupf N, Costa R, Luchsinger J, Tang MX, Lee JH, Mayeux R. "Relationship between plasma lipids and all-cause mortality in nondemented elderly." *J Am Geriatr Soc* 2005; 53 (2): 219-26.

50. Weverling-Rijnsburger AW, Jonkers IJ, van Exel E, Gussekloo J, Westendorp RG. "High-density vs low-density lipoprotein cholesterol as the risk factor for coronary artery disease and stroke in old age." *Arch Intern Med* 2003; 163 (13): 1549-54.

51. Upmeier E, Lavonius S, Lehtonen A, Viitanen M, Isoaho H, Arve S. "Serum lipids and their association with mortality in the elderly: a prospective cohort study." *Aging Clin Exp Res* 2009; 21 (6): 424-30.

52. Kwiterovich PO, Gidding SS. "Universal screening of cholesterol in children." Clin Cardiol 2012; 35 (11): 662-4.

53. Oliveira FL, Patin RV, Escrivao MA. "Atherosclerosis prevention and treatment in children and adolescents." *Expert Rev Cardiovasc Ther* 2010; 8 (4): 513-28.

54. Valsta LM, Tapanainen H, Sundvall J, Laatkainen T, Mannisto S, Pietinen P, Vartiainen E. "Explaining the 25-year decline of serum cholesterol by dietary changes and use of lipid lowering medications in Finland." *Public Health Nutr* 2010;13 (6A): 932-8.

55. Pietinen P, Vartianen E, Seppanen R, Aro A, Puska P. "Changes in diet in Finland from 1972 to 1992: the impact on coronary heart disease risk." *Prev Med* 1996; 25 (3): 243-50.

CHAPTER 6

Paleo Favorites: Harmful or Healthful?

The Paleo diet appeals to beef lovers since it encourages red meat. Most Paleo meals are centered on meat, poultry, fish, or eggs. This sounds much like a standard meal in the United States. Who doesn't like the taste of a typical bacon-and-egg breakfast? It is no surprise then that so many people are attracted to this trendy diet. Paleo supporters also tend to promote game meat and grass-fed meat, such as bison and venison.

Paleo favorites include:

- Grass-fed beef
- Wild fish and game
- Eggs

Grass-Fed Beef

One of the supposed explanations for why it is OK to eat unrestricted amounts of meat is that the type of saturated fat in meat and eggs is stearic acid, which typically does not raise cholesterol. Specifically, grass-fed beef is touted for having more stearic acid than regular beef.[1] While stearic acid is not as dangerous as palmitic acid,[2] it is actually not the main saturated fat in most meat, even grass-fed beef.[3]

The main saturated fat in both regular beef and grass-fed beef is palmitic acid.[3] In fact, nearly all common animal products have palmitic acid as their *main* saturated fat with stearic in a *smaller* proportion.[3] Palmitic acid is worse than stearic acid because it raises LDL (bad) cholesterol more without raising HDL (good) cholesterol as much as other saturated fat.[2]

Though grass-fed beef is lower in total fat when compared with regular beef, the main saturated fat in both is still palmitic acid.[3] The saturated fat in grass-fed beef is 56% palmitic and 34% stearic, while regular beef has similar proportions with 59% palmitic and 32% stearic.[3] Butter and bacon are particularly high in saturated fat, but cheese and milk are also rich in the same kind of fat. Chicken has a particularly high proportion of palmitic acid to stearic acid. All of these foods, however, are rich in palmitic acid. (See the table below for the types of fat in animal products.)

Type of Saturated Fat (in Grams) in Animal Products

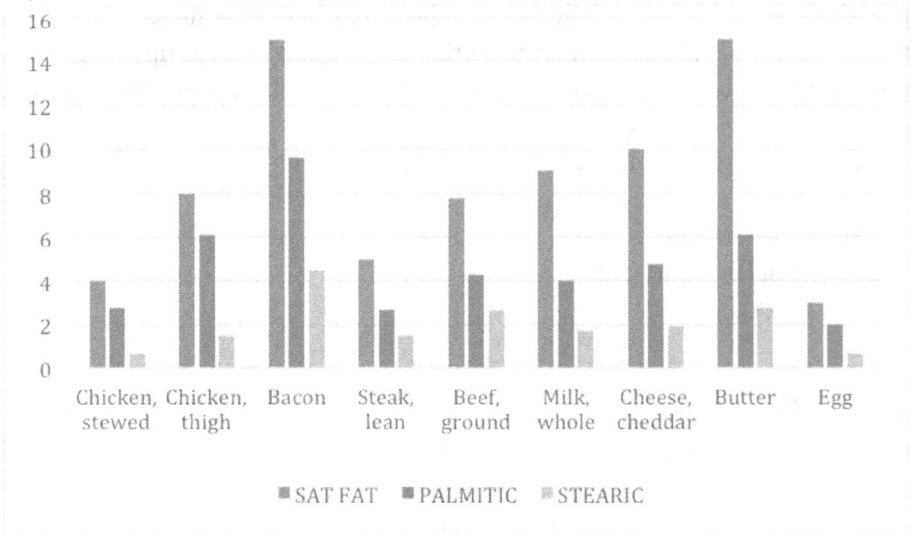

Data compiled by Jen Swallow from US Department of Agriculture, Agricultural Research Service. 2014. USDA National Nutrient Database for Standard Reference, Release 27. Nutrient Data Laboratory home page, http://www.ars.usda.gov/nutrientdata.

Wild Fish and Game

Just as grass-fed beef is believed to be healthier than regular beef, wild game is promoted for its health benefits by Paleo enthusiasts. What can be more illustrative of our Paleolithic ancestors than a man hunting wild animals or fishing? Modern hunters enjoy game meat such as venison, bison, and reindeer, much like cavemen enjoyed eating wild game.

But does game meat actually have health benefits? Does it affect blood cholesterol in a different way than regular beef does? Is it heart healthy? In 2013, Swedish researchers compared blood samples from a group of participants who regularly ate reindeer (game) with a group eating non-game meat.[4] In the game-meat group, a majority, 65%, had high cholesterol (greater than or equal to 240 mg/dL) compared with the group eating nongame meat, in which 38% had high cholesterol.[4] Additionally, game-meat eaters did not have a lower incidence of heart disease than regular meat eaters in nearby regions.[4] Game meat, therefore, does not appear to be heart healthy. This makes sense after seeing how grass-fed meat is rich in palmitic acid, which raises cholesterol.[2, 3]

Another reason to limit consumption of game meat is heavy-metal contamination.[5-7] Particles of heavy metals are commonly found in the air, soil, and water. These metals accumulate with each step up the food chain, particularly in the organs of animals. Wild animals tend to experience this accumulation much like farm animals. This kind of contamination can happen with red meat, fish, or seafood. Internal organs, such as liver, tend to accumulate heavy metals such as lead and cadmium. Predatory fish, such as swordfish and tuna, also tend to accumulate heavy metals.

In some populations that frequently eat game meat and organs, blood levels of lead are associated with game-meat intake, while mercury is linked to fish and seafood intake.[5, 6] Cadmium and arsenic, two toxic substances, are also reflected in blood tests by seafood intake.[6] Lead, mercury, cadmium, and arsenic are all potentially toxic substances. Lead can be toxic for the brain and kidneys when blood levels go above recommended values.[5] Cadmium can be toxic to the liver and kidneys.[8, 9]

Other toxic contaminants, such as dioxin, PCBs, and PFAs, are commonly found in meat.[10-13] PFAs are chemicals used to produce nonstick cookware, flame retardants, and plastic wrappers. Though these toxins are found in plant foods as well, the levels are higher in fish and meat. PFAs are toxic to the brain and can accumulate in the body.[13, 14] One study of over 80,000 participants showed an increased risk of congenital cerebral palsy with high levels of PFAs in pregnant women.[14]

Fish and seafood are major dietary sources of these pollutants, but game meat is also a significant contributor.[9-13] This is likely due to the concentration of contaminants that occurs in the food chain where plants are at the bottom and animals are closer to the top. Milk and dairy can also be major dietary sources of dioxins and PCBs.[10, 11]

What about game meat compared with meat from a farm? Farmed animals also have heavy-metal contamination, though the levels in muscle tissue are generally lower than those of internal organs. The other important factor to consider in this comparison is the type of ammunition used to hunt, since lead ammunition can contaminate game meat. Meat from a factory farm has direct exposure to other contaminants, such as antibiotics and pesticide residues from feed.[15]

Both types of meat have their drawbacks. Beef and chicken from farms often have detectable residues of antibiotics.[15-18] Despite the absence of antibiotics, growth hormones, and pesticide residues, game meat should not be considered a health food to be eaten every day. Eating a serving of game meat once a month or even once a week may not be harmful, but eating it twice a day or once a day could cause health issues.

Eggs

Are eggs truly incredible? Should we eat eggs every day? The egg has been promoted then demonized so many times, yet many still believe eggs are a health food. Why was the egg ever considered evil? After all, it is so rich in protein and vitamins!

Good Eggs

Protein is made of amino acids, some of which are essential and some of which are nonessential. "Essential" means that the body cannot make adequate amounts of this substance, while "nonessential" means that the body can make enough for good health. A "complete" protein has all nine of the essential amino acids: threonine, lysine, leucine, isoleucine, histidine, methionine, tryptophan, valine, and phenylalanine. Though both animal products, such as eggs, and plant foods, such as lentils, have all of the essential amino acids, some have more than others.

Eggs have a good balance of the essential amino acids, which make them a popular source of complete protein. Eggs, therefore, have a high-quality protein because quality is associated with the relative amounts of essential amino acids. But do eggs have more of a complete protein than other foods? In other words, is the *kind* of protein in eggs far superior to that of other foods?

Surprisingly, the answer is not necessarily. Although egg protein is slightly higher in total essential amino acids, it has a similar balance of essential amino acids when compared with many other foods.[3] Looking at each essential amino acid, other animal and plant foods have amounts close to those of the egg.[3] Eggs have about 9 g of essential amino acids in 20 grams of total protein, which means that over half of the protein in eggs is nonessential.[3] In comparison, chicken and beef have closer to 8 g of essential amino acids in 20 g of total protein, which is what numerous plant foods have as well.[3]

The quality of animal protein is therefore similar to, but not necessarily superior to, the quality of plant protein. Each food has different amounts of essential amino acids. Eggs are particularly high in threonine and valine, for example.[3] Eggs have more of those amino acids than many other popular foods.[3] Compared with eggs, on the other hand, chia seeds and sesame seeds have more methionine, and tofu has more tryptophan in 20 g of total protein.[3]

Popular plant protein foods are not missing or totally lacking any one particular essential amino acid.[3] They simply have more of some and less of other essential amino acids when compared with animal proteins. But there is no need to worry about getting a methionine deficiency or deficiency in any other amino acid because it is simply implausible. Protein deficiency does not usually happen without a general deficiency in total calories. When a variety of foods are eaten throughout one day, it is very easy to get enough complete proteins even from exclusively plant foods. (See the graph of complete protein foods below. The foods in this graph contain both essential and nonessential amino acids. Only the essential amino acids are presented. It takes roughly ½ cup to 2 cups of food to get 20 g of protein, depending on which food is chosen. Data in this graph are compiled from the USDA National Nutrient Database.)

Estimated Essential Amino Acids in Protein Foods

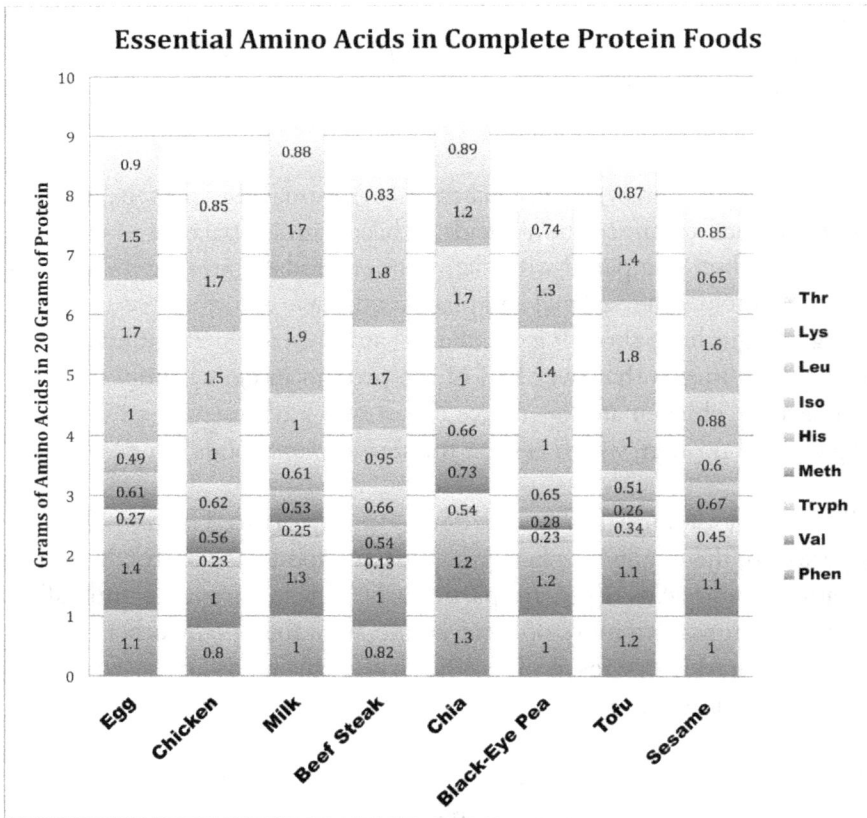

Essential Amino Acids in Complete Protein Foods

Y-axis: Grams of Amino Acids in 20 Grams of Protein (0 to 10)

Legend: Thr, Lys, Leu, Iso, His, Meth, Tryph, Val, Phen

Data values by food (bottom to top):

Food	Phen	Val	Tryph	Meth	His	Iso	Leu	Lys	Thr
Egg	1.1	1.4	0.27	0.61	0.49	1	1.7	1.5	0.9
Chicken	0.8	1, 0.23	0.56	0.62	1	1.5	1.7	0.85	
Milk	1	1.3	0.25	0.53	0.61	1	1.9	1.7	0.88
Beef Steak	0.82	1, 0.13	0.54	0.66	0.95	1.7	1.8	0.83	
Chia	1.3	1.2	0.54	0.73	0.66	1	1.7	1.2	0.89
Black-Eye Pea	1	1.2	0.23	0.28	0.65	1	1.4	1.3	0.74
Tofu	1.2	1.1	0.34	0.26	0.51	1	1.8	1.4	0.87
Sesame	1	1.1	0.45	0.67	0.6	0.88	1.6	0.65	0.85

Data compiled by Jen Swallow from US Department of Agriculture, Agricultural Research Service. 2014. USDA National Nutrient Database for Standard Reference, Release 27. Nutrient Data Laboratory home page, http://www.ars.usda.gov/nutrientdata.

Bad Eggs

Along with protein, eggs have several other components. For instance, eggs are the most concentrated source of cholesterol when compared with any other popular American food. One large egg has 186 mg of cholesterol.[3] More than three eggs are needed to get 20 g of protein,[3] which come with 550 mg of cholesterol.[3] (See *Cholesterol, Fat, and Fiber in Select Foods* graph for cholesterol found in 20 g of protein from different foods.)

Cholesterol, Fat, and Fiber in Select Foods

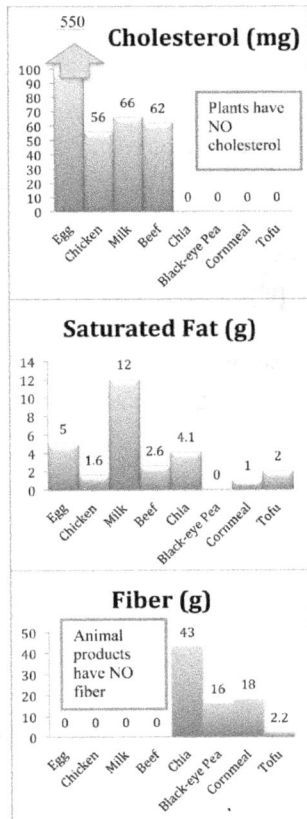

Data compiled by Jen Swallow from US Department of Agriculture, Agricultural Research Service. 2014. USDA National Nutrient Database for Standard Reference, Release 27. Nutrient Data Laboratory home page, http://www.ars.usda.gov/nutrientdata.

One egg does not have a great deal of saturated fat, but an omelet made of three eggs, for example, has more saturated fat than a serving of beef.[3] To make matters worse, eggs—just like other animal products—do not have any fiber. (See the *Cholesterol, Fat, and Fiber in Select Foods* graphs for sat fat/fiber found in 20 g of protein from different foods.)

Is eating cholesterol harmless? Does dietary cholesterol actually influence blood cholesterol? Low-carb advocates often think that it is completely harmless, much like they believe that saturated fat is harmless.[4] Even the new US dietary guidelines are removing a restriction on dietary cholesterol, so it is no wonder that people continue to believe it is of no major concern.

In reality, saturated fat intake has a stronger effect than cholesterol on blood lipids in general. This may be due to the fact that we eat much more saturated fat (in grams) than we do cholesterol (in milligrams). Eating cholesterol, however, does usually increase blood cholesterol.[19-31] Neither one is benign when consumed in excess, especially in the context of a low-fiber and low-carb diet.

How, then, did the whole idea originate about cholesterol being benign? The fact is that some people respond differently than do others to dietary cholesterol.[27] When it comes to cholesterol, people generally fall into two categories: hyper-responders and hyporesponders.[27] Eating cholesterol raises blood cholesterol significantly more in hyper-responders, while it only raises it a small bit in hyporesponders.[27]

So how do you know if you are a hyper-responder or hyporesponder? Ask your doctor for a lipid panel if you have been eating eggs every day and look at the results, then continue the same exact diet without any eggs for two months and get another lipid panel. If your cholesterol level dropped significantly after removing eggs from your diet and you did not lose weight, then you may be a hyper-responder. (Weight loss can drop cholesterol levels and confound the results of the test.)

Even in healthy populations, more than one in four people are hyperresponders.[33] But hyporesponders may not be immune to the effects of eating eggs, especially if they have diabetes. Consuming an egg a day doubles the risk of heart disease in diabetics and people who develop diabetes later in life.[32] Even if you are a hyporesponder, make sure to check your HbA1c level each year at the doctor's office to monitor diabetes risk.

Reviewing a combination of ten new and old studies, eating cholesterol consistently raised cholesterol in women and men.[19-31] Many healthy adults may respond mildly or not at all to dietary cholesterol,[33] but on average, an egg or more per day is more likely to raise cholesterol than to have no effect.[19-31] The fact remains that Americans do not eat as much cholesterol as those on a low-carb diet. The average American does not eat more than one large egg per day.[34] If they did, it would mean a total cholesterol intake of over 400 mg.[3, 34]

On a gluten-free, low-carb diet like Paleo, eggs are frequently on the menu since there is no cereal, oatmeal, or toast for breakfast. Having a Paleo-style breakfast with three or four eggs every day may not be the best idea as it can total over 500 mg of cholesterol. There is a big difference between eating eggs as a weekend treat and making them the center of every meal.

The association between cholesterol intake and heart disease risk is about a 6% increase in risk for 200 mg/1,000 calories per day.[20] Eating several eggs per day in addition to other animal proteins, such as meat and cheese, can drastically affect the risk for heart disease and diabetes.[35-47] Though dietary cholesterol affects people differently, it tends to have a negative effect when consumed in excess.[35-47] (See the *Eggs and Cholesterol* table for studies on how egg intake affects blood cholesterol.)

Eggs and Cholesterol

Year	Country	Author	Subject #	Length/ Test	Results
2013	USA	Baumgar tner et al [22]	117	3 mo	Total cholesterol increased by 24 mg/dL and LDL increased by 22 mg/dL in women eating 1 egg/day (in addition to the 1 egg/wk regular intake)
2013	Turkey	Golzar et al [23]	4	30 days	LDL cholesterol increased and HDL decreased in men eating 1 egg/day
2013	USA	Blesso et al [24]	37	3 mo	HDL and large LDL particles increased while small LDL particles decreased in patients with metabolic syndrome eating 3 eggs/day
2012	Canada	Spence et al [25]	1262	Duplex Ultrasou nd	Carotid plaque area was 125 +/- 129 mm in patients eating <2 eggs/wk and 132+/- 142 mm in those eating 3 or more eggs/wk.
2006	Brazil	Cesar et al [26]	25	2 wk	Eating 3 eggs/day increased LDL and HDL cholesterol in healthy men
2002	USA	Herron et al [27]	51	30 days	Eating 1 egg/day increased total cholesterol in some healthy women but not others
1997	USA	Knopp et al [28]	161	3 mo	Eating 2 eggs/day increased LDL by 3 mg/dL in patients with mildly high cholesterol and 12 mg/dL in patients with high triglycerides.
1994	USA	Ginsberg et al [29]	20	2 mo	Eating 1 egg/day increased total cholesterol by 3 mg/dL in young healthy men
1995	USA	Ginsberg et al [30]	13	2 mo	Eating 1 egg/day increased LDL by 5 mg/dL and HDL increased by 1 mg/dL in women
1987	USA	Zanni et al [31]	9	2 wk	For 745 mg of egg cholesterol , the number of LDL particles increased by 17%, particle size also increased.

In 2008, Harvard Medical School researchers studied 21,000 people and discovered a positive relationship between egg intake and mortality, though it did not specifically raise heart attack or stroke risk for nondiabetics.[35] Participants in this study had a median intake of a single egg per week, so this may explain why the relationship was not significant for heart disease. When the egg intake shot up to one or more every day, there was a significant increase in the risk of early death.[35] The risk of death for diabetic subjects was twofold when the lowest intake was compared with the highest intake of eggs: from less than one per week to one or more per day.[35]

Scientists at the University of North Carolina found that egg consumption was not associated with cardiovascular disease (CVD) risk, but it may increase the incidence of type 2 diabetes among the general population and CVD risk in diabetic patients.[35] CVD includes heart disease, stroke, heart failure, and heart valve problems. Compared with those who never eat eggs, those who eat an egg or more per day are 42% more likely to develop type 2 diabetes.[35] Among diabetics, frequent egg-eaters are 69% more likely to have heart disease.[35]

In 2013, scientists in China reviewed data from fourteen studies on 320,000 subjects, which showed a dose-response association between egg consumption and the risk of CVD and diabetes.[38] This analysis measured intake by increment doses of four eggs per week.[38] Again, they found that eating eggs was more dangerous for diabetics.[38]

(See *Eggs, Disease, and Mortality* table for studies on how egg intake affects disease and mortality.)

Eggs, Disease, and Mortality

Year	Country	Author	Subject #	Type	Results
2014	International	Tran et al[35]	400,000	Review	Half of the studies showed a link between diabetes and egg intake.
2013	USA	Shin et al[36]	90,000	Meta-Analysis	Eating 1 egg/day was not significantly associated with CVD but it was linked to type 2 diabetes in the general population and CVD in diabetics.
2013	China	Rong et al[37]	400,000	Meta-Analysis	Eating up to 1 egg/day is not linked to heart disease or stroke in healthy subjects but is linked to heart disease among diabetics.
2013	International	Li et al[38]	320,000	Meta-Analysis	There is a dose-response positive relationship between egg intake, the risk of CVD and diabetes.
2012	Lithuania	Radzevecene et al[39]	234	Case-Control	Eating >5 eggs/wk resulted in a 3-fold increased risk of type 2 diabetes.
2011	USA	Houston et al[40]	1,941	Cohort	High dietary cholesterol and egg consumption was associated with a 1.5-fold increased risk of CVD in the entire cohort and 3-fold risk for diabetics.
2011	China	Shi et al[41]	2,800	Qualitative	Triglycerides and total cholesterol was higher in women eating >2eggs/wk vs less. Egg intake was linked to diabetes risk in women.
2008	USA	Djousse et al[42]	21,000	Cohort	Eating ≥1egg/day was positively related to overall mortality in general and a 2-fold increased risk for diabetics.
2007	USA	Qureshi et al[43]	9,700	Cohort	Eating 1 egg/day was not linked to heart disease in non-diabetics but did increase risk in diabetics.
2006	Japan	Nakamur et al[44]	90,000	Cohort	Eating 1 egg/day was not linked to heart disease but total cholesterol intake was.
2004	Japan	Nakamur et al[45]	9,000	Cohort	Total cholesterol was related to egg consumption. All-cause mortality was lower in women eating 2 eggs/wk vs 1 egg/day.
1999	USA	Hu et al[46]	110,000	Cohort	Eating 1 egg/day was not related to heart disease in non-diabetics but increased risk in diabetics.

The Egg Conclusion

In the United States, where heart disease is the top killer,[47] and 40% of the population has prediabetes or diabetes,[48] everyone should consider shifting to a heart-healthy diet. In the past three decades, the prevalence of diabetes has doubled among all age groups.[48] Diabetes now affects one in five Americans above the age of sixty-five.[48] Diabetics are at an increased risk of dying from heart disease. The government could save an unimaginable amount of money from health-care costs alone if everyone switched to a heart-healthy diet. As other countries shift to a Western diet, they start to experience the same health problems. In China, for instance, the prevalence of prediabetes is 50%, and many cases of full-blown diabetes remain undiagnosed.[49]

Whether people are hyper- or hyporesponders to dietary cholesterol, focusing on high-fiber foods along with plant protein can only benefit health. Eating more than one egg a day, on the other hand, may increase the risk of diabetes in the general population.[36] Some people might even get away with eating up to one egg each day without increasing the risk of heart disease, but why not stay on the safe side?

For those who desire eggs, cutting down to two eggs on the weekend as a treat is probably wise. This two-egg-per-week maximum can help, especially if you have any risk factors for diabetes or heart disease like obesity, sedentary lifestyle, or a family history of these diseases. Most adults do not need the extra protein because they are already getting enough. Even older nondiabetic adults may benefit from eating no more than four eggs per week.[50]

Cholesterol is not an essential dietary nutrient. The human body actually makes enough of its own cholesterol.[51] Many individuals survive and thrive purely on plant foods, which means they are not eating any cholesterol. The fact is that clogged arteries contain cholesterol deposits among other components,[47] so eating more cholesterol and fat can be counterproductive, especially in the presence of chronic inflammation. Fat and cholesterol should move quickly through blood vessels, and eating several eggs may impair that movement.[26] Clogged arteries are not only a sign of heart disease but also of stroke, peripheral artery disease, chronic kidney disease, and coronary microvascular disease.[47]

I often see several such diagnoses in medical charts at my work. Some patients with these diseases have no symptoms until a stroke or heart attack occurs,[47] and then it may be too late to diagnose the illness. An effective method to lower the risk of heart disease is to eat foods known to lower blood cholesterol, which is why dietary recommendations have long focused on eating more fiber, less saturated fat, *and* less cholesterol.

Notes:

1. "Why Grass-Fed Trumps Grain-Fed", Chris Kresser, Accessed February 25, 2015, http://chriskresser.com/why-grass-fed-trumps-grain-fed/.
2. Micha R, Mozaffarian D. "Saturated fat and cardiometabolic risk factors, coronary heart disease, stroke, and diabetes: a fresh look at the evidence." *Lipids* 2010; 45 (10): 893-905.
3. U.S. Department of Agriculture, Agricultural Research Service. 2014. USDA National Nutrient Database for Standard Reference, Release 27. Nutrient Data Laboratory Home Page, Accessed February 25, 2015, http://www.ars.usda.gov/nutrientdata.
4. "Why Cholesterol is Not Bad", Sébastien Noël, Accessed March 8, 2015, http://paleoleap.com/cholesterol-is-not-bad/
5. Igl W, Kamal Eldin A, Johansson A, Liebisch G, Gnewuch C, Schmitz G, Gyllensten U. "Animal source food intake and association with blood cholesterol, glycerophospholipids and shingolipids in a northern Swedish population." *Int J Circumpolar Health* 2013; 72.
6. Bjermo H, Sand S, Nalsen C, Lundh T, Enghardt Barbieri H, Pearson M, et al. "Lead, mercury, and cadmium in blood and their relation to diet among Swedish adults." *Food Chem Toxicol* 2013; 57: 161-9.
7. Birgisdottir BE, Knutsen HK, Haugen M, Gjelstad IM, Jennsen MT, Ellingsen DG, et al. "Essential and toxic element concentrations

in blood and urine and their associations with diet: results from a Norwegian population study including high-consumers of seafood and game." *Sci Total Environ* 2013; 463-464: 836-44.

8. Lazarus M, Prevendar Crnic A, Bilandzic N, Kusak J, Reljiic S. "Cadmium, lead, and mercury exposure assessment among Croatian consumers of free-living game." *Arh Hig Rada Toksikol* 2014; 65 (3): 281-92.

9. Matovic V, Buha A, Dukic-Cosic D, Bulat Z. "Insight into the oxidative stress induced by lead and/or cadmium in blood, liver, and kidneys." *Food Chem Toxicol* 2015. [Epub ahead of print.]

10. Wong WW, Yip YC, Choi KK, Ho YY, Xiao Y. "Dietary exposure to dioxins and dioxin-like PCBs of Hong Kong adults: results of the first Hong Kong Total Diet Study." *Food Addit Contam Part A Chem Anal Control Expo Risk Assess*. 2013; 30 (12): 2152-8.

11. Mihats D, Moche W, Prean M, Rauscher-Gabernig E. "Dietary exposure to non-dioxin-like PCBs of different population groups in Austria." *Chemosphere* 2015; 126C: 53-59.

12. Rauscher-Gabernig E, Mischek D, Moche W, Prean M. "Dietary intake of dioxins, furans and dioxin-like PCBs in Austria." *Food Addit Contam Part A Chem Anal Control Expo Risk Assess* 2013; 30 (10): 1770-9.

13. Berg V, Nost TH, Huber S, Rylander C, Hansen S, Veyhe AS, et al. "Maternal serum concentrations of per- and polyfluoroalkyl substances and their predictors in years with reduced production and use." *Environ Int* 2014; 69: 58-66.

14. Liew Z, Ritz B, Bonefeld-Jorgensen EC, Henriksen TB, Nohr EA, Bech BH, et al. "Prenatal exposure to perfluoroalkyl substances and the risk of congenital cerebral palsy in children." *Am J Epid* 2014; 180 (6): 574-581.

15. Schneider MJ, Yun L, Lehotay SJ. "Terbium-sensitised luminescence screening method for fluoroquinolones in beef serum." *Food Addit Contam Part A Chem Anal Control Expo Risk Assess* 2013; 30 (4): 666-9.

16. Reyes-Herrera I, Donoghue DJ. "Antibiotic residues distribute uniformly in broiler chicken breast muscle tissue." *J Food Prot* 2008; 71 (1): 223-5.

17. Reyes-Herrera I, Schneider MJ, Blore PJ, Donoghue DJ. "The relationship between blood and muscle samples to monitor for residues of the antibiotic enrofloxacin in chickens." *Poult Sci* 2011; 90 (2): 481-5.
18. Dey BP, Thaker NH, Bright SA, Thaler AM. "Fast antimicrobial screen test (FAST): improved screen test for detecting antimicrobial residues in meat tissue." *J AOAC Int* 2005; 88 (2): 447-54.
19. Levy Y, Maor I, Presser D, Aniram M. "Consumption of eggs in meals increase the susceptibility of human plasma and low-density lipoprotein to lipid peroxidation." *Ann Nutr Metab* 1996; 40 (5): 243-51.
20. Kritchevsky SB, Kritchevsky D. "Egg consumption and coronary heart disease: an epidemiological overview." *J Am Coll Nutr* 2000; 19 (5Suppl) 549s-555s.
21. Severins N, Mensink RP, Plat J. "Effects of lutein-enriched egg yolk in buttermilk or skimmed milk on serum lipids & lipoproteins of mildly hypercholesterolemic subjects." *Nutr Metab Cardiovasc Dis* 2014. [Epub ahead of print.]
22. Baumgartner S, Kelly ER, van der Made S, Berendschot TT, Husche C, Lutjohann D. "The influence of consuming an egg or an egg-yolk buttermilk drink for 12 wk on serum lipids, inflammation, and liver function markers in human volunteers." *Nutrition* 2013; 29 (10): 1237-44.
23. Golzar Adabi SH, Ahbab M, Fani AR, Halibabaei A, Cevian N, Cooper RG. "Egg yolk fatty acid profile of avian species—influence on human nutrition." *J Anim Physiol Anim Nutr (Berl)* 2013; 97 (1): 27-38.
24. Blesso CN, Anderson CJ, Barona J, Volek JS, Fernandez ML. "Whole egg consumption improves lipoprotein profiles and insulin sensitivity to a greater extent than yolk-free egg substitute in individuals with metabolic syndrome." *Metabolism* 2013; 62 (3): 400-10.
25. Spence JD, Jenkins DJ, Davignon J. "Egg yolk consumption and carotid plaque." *Atherosclerosis* 2012; 224 (2): 469-73.
26. Cesar TB, Oliveira MR, Mesquita CH, Maranhao RC. "High cholesterol intake modifies chylomicron metabolism in normolipidemic young men." *J Nutr* 2006; 136 (4): 971-6.

27. Herron KL, Vega-Lopez S, Conde K, Ramjiganesh T, Roy S, Shachter NS, Fernandez ML. "Pre-menopausal women, classified as hypo- or hyperresponders, do not alter their LDL/HDL ratio following a high dietary cholesterol challenge." *J Am Coll Nutr* 2002; 21 (3): 250-8.

28. Knopp RH, Retzlaff BM, Walden CE, Dowdy AA, Tsunehara CH, Austin MA, et al. "A double-blind, randomized, controlled trial of the effects of two eggs per day in moderately hypercholesterolemic and combined hyperlipidemic subjects taught the NCEP step 1 diet." *J Am Coll Nutr* 1997; 16 (6): 551-61.

29. Ginsberg HN, Karmally W, Siddiqui M, Hollerand S, Tall AR, Rumsey SC, et al. "A dose-response study of the effects of dietary cholesterol on fasting and postprandial lipid and lipoprotein metabolism in healthy young men." *Arteriosclerosis Thromb* 1994; 14 (4): 576-86.

30. Ginsberg HN, Karmaliv W, Siddiqui M, Holleran S, Tall AR, Blaner WS, et al. "Increase in dietary cholesterol are associated with modest increases in both LDL and HDL cholesterol in healthy young women." *Arteriosclerosis Thromb Vasc Biol* 1995; 15 (2): 169-78.

31. Zanni EE, Zannis VI, Blum CB, Herbert PN, Breslow JL. "Effect of egg cholesterol and dietary fats on plasma lipids, lipoproteins, and apoproteins of normal women consuming natural diets." *J Lipids Res* 1987; 28 (5): 518-27.

32. Spence JD, Jenkins DJ, Davignon J. "Dietary cholesterol and egg yolks: not for patients at risk of vascular disease." *Can J Cardiol* 2010; 26 (9): e336-9.

33. Fernandez ML. "Dietary cholesterol provided by eggs and plasma lipoproteins in healthy populations." *Curr Opin Clin Nutr Metab Care* 2006; 9 (1): 8-12.

34. "What We Eat in America", NHANES 2011-2012, Accessed March 30, 2015, http://www.ars.usda.gov/SP2UserFiles/Place/80400530/pdf/1112/Table_1_NIN_GEN_11.pdf.

35. Tran NL, Barraj LM, Hellman JM, Scrafford CG. "Egg consumption and cardiovascular disease among diabetic individuals: a systemic review of the literature." *Diabetes Metab Syndr Obes* 2014; 7: 121-37.

36. Shin JY, Xun P, Nakamura Y, He K. "Egg consumption in relation to risk of cardiovascular disease and diabetes: a systematic review and meta-analysis." *Am J Clin Nutr* 2013; 98 (1): 146-59.

37. Rong Y, Chen L, Zhu T, Song Y, Yu M, Shan Z, et al. "Egg consumption and risk of coronary heart disease and stroke: a dose-response meta-analysis of prospective cohort studies." *BMJ* 2013; 346: e8539.

38. Li Y, Zhou C, Zhou X, Li L. "Egg consumption and risk of cardiovascular diseases and diabetes: a meta-analysis." *Atherosclerosis* 2013; 229 (2): 524-30.

39. Radzeviciene L, Ostrauskas R. "Egg consumption and the risk of type 2 diabetes mellitus: a case-control study." *Public Health Nutr* 2012; 15 (8): 1437-41.

40. Houston DK, Ding J, Lee JS, Garcia M, Kanaya AM, Tylavsky FA, Newman AB, Visser M, Kritchevsky SB; Health ABC Study. "Dietary fat and cholesterol and risk of cardiovascular disease in older adults: the Health ABC Study." *Nutr Metab Cardiovasc Dis.* 2011 Jun; 21 (6): 430-7.

41. Shi Z, Yuan B, Zhang C, Zhou M, Holmboe-Ottesen G. "Egg consumption and risk of diabetes in adults, Jiangsu, China." *Nutrition* 2011; 27 (2): 194-8.

42. Djousse L, Gaziano JM. "Egg consumption in relation to cardiovascular disease mortality: the Physicians' Health Study." *Am J Clin Nutr* 2008; 87 (4): 964-9.

43. Qureshi AI, Suri FK, Ahmed S, Nesar A, Divani AA, Kirmani JF. "Regular egg consumption does not increase the risk of stroke and cardiovascular diseases." *Med Sci Monit* 2007; 13 (1): CR1-8.

44. Nakamura Y, Iso H, Kita Y, Ueshima H, Okada K, Konishi M, et al. "Egg consumption, serum total cholesterol concentrations and coronary heart disease incidence: Japan Public Health Center-based prospective study." *Br J Nutr* 2006; 96 (5): 921-8.

45. Nakamura Y, Okamura T, Tamaki S, Kadowaki T, Hayaki T, Kita Y, et al. "Egg consumption, serum cholesterol, and cause-specific and all-cause mortality: the National Integrated Project for Prospective Observation of Non-communicable Disease and its Trends in the

Aged, 1980 (NIPPON DATA80)." *Am J Clin Nutr* 2004; 80 (1): 58-63.

46. Hu FB, Stampfer MJ, Rimm EB, Manson JE, Ascherio A, Colditz GA, et al. "A prospective study of egg consumption and risk of cardiovascular disease in men and women." *JAMA* 1999; 281 (15): 1387-94.

47. "What is Atherosclerosis", NIH, National Heart, Lung, and Blood Institute, Accessed September 5, 2015, http://www.nhlbi.nih.gov/health/health-topics/topics/atherosclerosis.

48. Cowie CC, Rust KF, Ford ES, Eberhardt MS, Byrd-Holt DD, Li C, et al. "Full accounting of diabetes and pre-diabetes in the U.S. population in 1988-1994 and 2005-2006." *Diabetes Care* 2009; 32 (2): 287-94.

49. Xu Y, Wang L, He J, Bi Y, Li M, Wang T, et al. "Prevalence and control of diabetes in Chinese adults." *JAMA* 2013; 310 (9): 948-59.

50. Virtanen JK, Mursu J, Tuomainen TP, Virtanen HE, Voutilainen S. "Egg consumption and risk of incident type 2 diabetes in men: the Kuopio Ischaemic Heart Disease Risk Factor Study[1,2,3]" 2015, doi:10.3945/ajcn.114.104109.

51. "Know Your Fats", American Heart Association, Accessed September 5, 2015, http://www.heart.org/HEARTORG/Conditions/Cholesterol/PreventionTreatmentofHighCholesterol/Know-Your-Fats_UCM_305628_Article.jsp.

52. "Your Guide to Lowering Your Cholesterol with TLC", US Department of Health and Human Services, NIH, National Heart, Lung, and Blood Institute, Accessed September 5, 2015, https://www.nhlbi.nih.gov/files/docs/public/heart/chol_tlc.pdf.

CHAPTER 7

Animal Protein versus Plant Protein

Protein is frequently hailed as a wonder nutrient in the media. The headlines say it can help you feel full, lose weight, heal faster, and build muscle. Despite all of this attention, major myths about this nutrient continue to propagate. Most people know that meat is high in protein, but they often do not realize that plants have protein too. A common myth is that plant protein is inferior in quality, or that we must combine different foods at the same meal to get a complete protein.

New research is piling up on the benefits of plant protein, yet the belief that humans need to eat meat daily to get enough protein is widespread. If humans need to eat meat every day to survive, then vegetarians would not live long. Likewise, if we need to eat meat to keep our muscles strong, then vegetarians would all be weak and puny. Vegans would be even worse off without meat, milk, or eggs. Indeed, a common misconception is that vegans are emaciated and deficient in several nutrients.

Vegetarians, therefore, can attest to the fact that protein is sorely misunderstood. Talk to vegetarians and find out what is the most common question people ask them. The answer is likely to be, "Where do you get your protein from?" Let's find out how, without meat or other animal products in every meal, we can find protein-rich options.

Protein in Common Foods

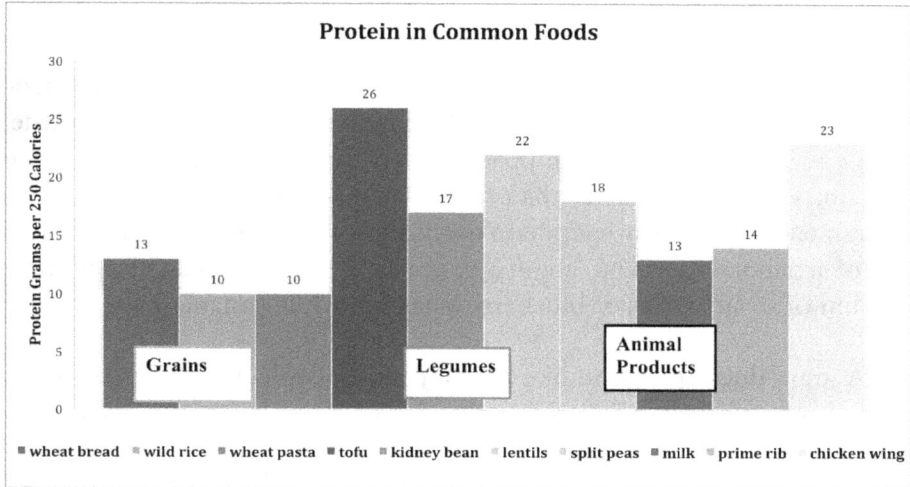

Protein in Common Foods

Y-axis: Protein Grams per 250 Calories (0, 5, 10, 15, 20, 25, 30)

Values: 13, 10, 10, 26, 17, 22, 18, 13, 14, 23

Categories: Grains, Legumes, Animal Products

Legend: wheat bread · wild rice · wheat pasta · tofu · kidney bean · lentils · split peas · milk · prime rib · chicken wing

The foods included above are examples of plant and animal proteins. Many different cuts and types of beef and chicken exist with varying amounts of protein. The beef included in this calculation is roasted prime rib, and the chicken is roasted chicken wing.[1]

Plants Have Enough Protein

Whole grains, beans, nuts, and seeds are all good sources of protein.[1] Does meat have more protein than beans or grains? Well, it depends on what kind of meat you are comparing to a given kind of grain or bean. Lean beef and poultry can have as much as 30 or 40 g of protein in a 6-oz portion.[1] Yes, it is true that lean meat has more protein per serving than most plant foods (see *Protein in Common Foods* graph), but it is usually not a dramatic difference when calories, fat, and fiber are taken into account.

In other cases, such as ground beef versus tofu, the amounts are very close. A cup of almonds has the same amount of protein as a cup of chopped chicken. A cup of whole wheat pasta has the same amount of protein as a cup of milk.[1] Two slices of whole wheat bread have as much protein as one egg.[1] Processed meats such as chicken nuggets, hot dogs, and sausage are lower in protein compared with plain chicken breast or steak. A cup of sausage has roughly the same amount of protein as a cup of lentils or split peas.[1]

To reinforce how misunderstood protein is, I have heard many people say that fruits and veggies have absolutely no protein. This is untrue. While produce is not high in protein, even fruits and veggies have some protein. Veggies are higher than fruit, but this does not mean that fruit has none. One cup of sweet potato or mushrooms has 4 g of protein, and a cup of artichoke hearts has about 5 g, nearly as much as an egg.[1] The same amount of strawberries or blueberries has 1 g, while bananas have 2 g.[1]

A gram does not sound like a lot for most people. On the other hand, for a short, thin lady who needs only 36 g of protein per day, every gram counts. In fact, there are some people who survive on a low-protein diet purely made of fruits. I do not recommend this kind of diet in the long term because of the low amounts of essential fatty acids, some vitamins, and minerals. In theory, a small fruitarian woman eating ten cups of bananas would get 20 g of total protein, which would still fall 16 g short of her needs. Simply adding two cups of beans to this diet brings the total up to her goal of 36 g. I still do not recommend this kind of diet, but it shows how adding beans, whole grains, and nuts to a plant-based diet would indeed provide sufficient protein.

You can easily get enough protein from plant foods as long as you eat enough. The major differences between animal and plant protein is not the quantity as much as the other nutrients that come along with the protein. Animal protein like beef, chicken, and eggs all have cholesterol, fat, no carbohydrates, and no fiber.[1] Whereas plant proteins, such as whole grains and beans, have carbohydrates, fiber, no cholesterol, and virtually no fat.[1] For this and many other reasons, vegetarians are often slimmer than meat eaters. Slim, however, does not necessarily mean weak.

Eating enough plant protein is pretty simple, even for those who do not eat meat. Complete proteins are those with all of the essential amino acids, which are not difficult to find in vegan or vegetarian diets.[2] When put to the test, vegans and vegetarians get a similar amount of essential amino acids in their diets and have similar amounts of muscle mass when compared with meat eaters (matched for the same BMI).[2]

Muscles Made from Plants

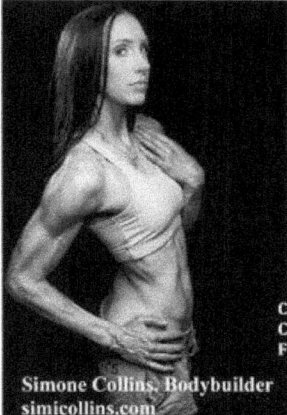

Simone Collins, Bodybuilder
simicollins.com
Facebook.com/simi.monique

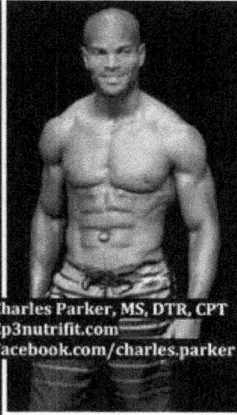

Charles Parker, MS, DTR, CPT
Cp3nutrifit.com
Facebook.com/charles.parker

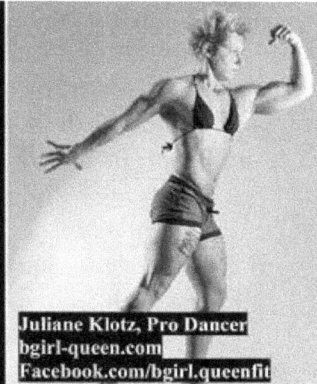

Juliane Klotz, Pro Dancer
bgirl-queen.com
Facebook.com/bgirl.queenfit

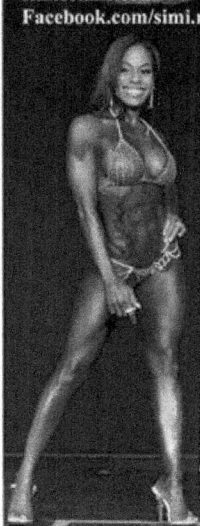

Cam F Awesome, Boxer
CamfAwesome.com
Facebook.com/Camfawesome

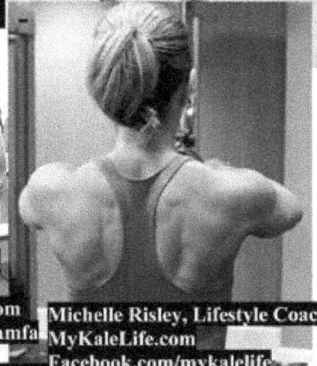

Michelle Risley, Lifestyle Coach
MyKaleLife.com
Facebook.com/mykalelife

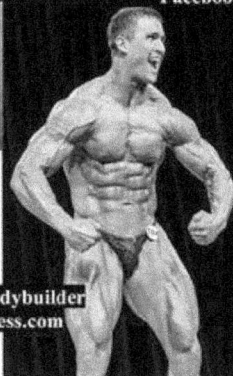

Luke Tan
Author, Bodybuilder
evolvedgeneration.com
Awakemethod.com

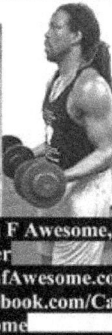

Harriet Davis , MD, Bodybuilder
mybikinimd.blogspot.com
veganbikinidoc.wordpress.com

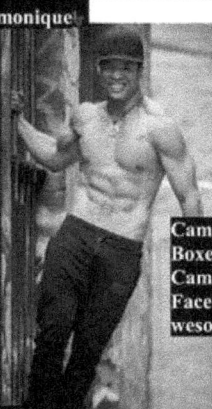

Ryan Nelson, Bodybuilder
RyanNelsonFitness.com

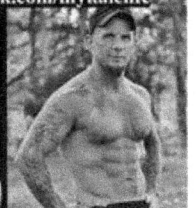

Aaron Macneil ,
Personal Trainer
AaronMacNeilsvegangrub.blogspot.com
instagram.com/veganshredit

Keep in mind that people who weigh more usually have more muscle even if they are obese. If you are normal weight, imagine carrying around a 60-lb barbell every day all day. Your body would have to adapt by growing more muscle tissue to carry this weight for so many hours. This can put a lot of dangerous pressure on joints and tendons, so I don't recommend buying a 60-lb barbell to try this experiment.

Long-time vegetarians tend to be normal weight, whereas the majority of American adults are overweight or obese. For this reason, subjects must be matched for BMI when comparing muscle mass. To illustrate this point, I compared myself with a friend who is the same height and weight as I am so we have the same BMI. When I measured her body fat, I noticed that she had 10% more fat that I do. This means that I have more muscle and less fat even though we weigh the same. In other words, just because people look thin, does not mean that they have low body fat.

Americans generally eat too much. Therefore, they can benefit from eating less total food, less fat, and more fiber. Vegetarians and vegans, on the other hand, tend to eat fewer total calories, less fat, less protein, and more fiber.[2] In general, eating enough protein to maintain muscle mass is not difficult. Meeting protein needs is as easy as eating enough food to meet energy needs, and most adults in the United States have no problem with that. Just because vegans and vegetarians eat less fat and total calories does not mean that they do not get enough protein to maintain muscle.[2]

How Much Protein Do We Need?

Despite all of the controversy about protein, US and Canadian dietary guidelines estimate that most adults need 0.8 g per kilogram of body weight,[3] which translates to roughly 70 g of protein for a man who weighs 200 lb. Similarly, according to the CDC and the National Institutes of Health, adults need about 50–65 g of protein.[4-6] Elderly and sick people may need more protein than do healthy adults. On average, though, most of us eat much more protein than we need; women eat about 70 g of protein with a total of 1,800 calories, and men eat 100 g of protein with a total of 2,500 calories daily.[7] This means that women are eating about 20 more grams of protein and men are eating 35 more grams of protein than they actually need.

Essential Amino Acids

Should we be worried about eating a complete protein at every meal? Not necessarily, since most of the protein we need each day does not have to be a complete protein. In fact, the majority of our protein requirements can be made up of incomplete protein or nonessential amino acids. Of the 65 g of protein recommended, only about 11 must be from essential amino acids.[8] This means 83% of the protein we need is nonessential, and a mere 17% of our total protein intake must be from essential amino acids.[8] With the average intake between 70 g and 100 g, we are inevitably getting more complete protein than we need.

What happens to the extra protein that our bodies do not use? It turns into fat, just as any extra calories do, regardless of whether they are carb, fat, or protein calories.[4] If you eat 35 g of extra protein, then you are also eating 140 extra calories each day. This translates to putting on 14 lb of body fat every year. This extra weight is simply from the excess protein that people eat, and it does not count the other excess calories from fat and sugar that may translate to even more body fat each year.

The bottom line is that plants have all the protein you need, no matter how big or tall you are. Are these proteins complete? Complete protein simply means a protein that contains all of the essential amino acids in a good balance to meet our nutrient needs. A common myth is that plant proteins are missing one or more essential amino acids and are therefore not complete. This is untrue. Plant protein foods contain all nine essential amino acids.[1]

Essential Amino Acid Recommended Intake[8] (g)	
Histidine	1.4
Isoleucine	1.1
Leucine	1.6
Lysine	1.4
Methionine	1.5
Threonine	0.8
Tryptophan	0.4
Valine	1.2.
Phenylalanine	1.6
Total	11

For example, plant proteins are not missing the amino acid methionine.[1] Sesame seeds and quinoa are good sources of methionine with 120% and 81%, respectively, of the same amount found in beef.[1] Grains are supposedly lacking lysine, yet oats and quinoa have about 60% of the lysine found in chicken.[1] Oats have more leucine, valine, phenylalanine, and tryptophan than chicken (comparing grams of total protein).[1]

Overall, meat has less of some and more of other essential amino acids when compared with plant proteins.[1] Each food is slightly different than the next, even when comparing one kind of meat to another; they all have variable amounts of each amino acid. For instance, chicken has almost double the amount of tryptophan that is found in beef.[1] That is one reason why it is important to have a variety of different foods each day, regardless of whether you eat meat or not. But the fact remains that most people eat more protein than they need, which contributes to obesity.

One choice in particular, the chia seed, stands out among other plant proteins. It is higher in all of the essential amino acids than most animal products (in a gram-per-gram comparison of total protein).[1] Chia seeds have more methionine and tryptophan than beef or chicken.[1] Not only are chia seeds packed with quality protein, but they are also an excellent source of omega-3 essential fat and fiber.[1] For this reason, I eat chia seeds daily and include them in some of the recipes in the last chapter of the book. (See the *Estimated Essential Amino Acids in Select Foods* graph for essential amino acids in more complete protein foods.)

Estimated Essential Amino Acids in Select Foods

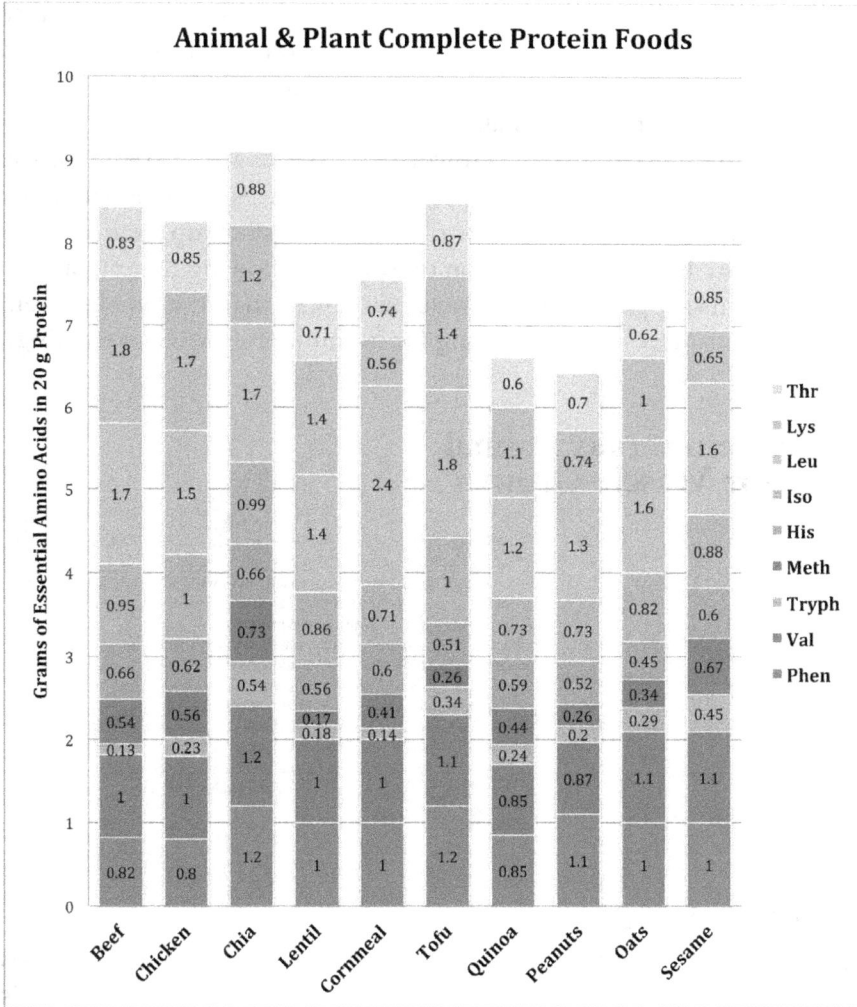

Animal & Plant Complete Protein Foods

Grams of Essential Amino Acids in 20 g Protein

Legend:
- Thr
- Lys
- Leu
- Iso
- His
- Meth
- Tryph
- Val
- Phen

Categories (x-axis): Beef, Chicken, Chia, Lentil, Cornmeal, Tofu, Quinoa, Peanuts, Oats, Sesame

Beef: 0.83, 1.8, 1.7, 0.95, 0.66, 0.54, 0.13, 1, 0.82

Chicken: 0.85, 1.7, 1.5, 1, 0.62, 0.56, 0.23, 1, 0.8

Chia: 0.88, 1.2, 1.7, 0.99, 0.66, 0.73, 0.54, 1.2, 1.2

Lentil: 0.71, 1.4, 1.4, 0.86, 0.56, 0.17, 0.18, 1, 1

Cornmeal: 0.74, 0.56, 2.4, 1.4, 0.71, 0.6, 0.41, 0.14, 1, 1

Tofu: 0.87, 1.4, 1.8, 1, 0.51, 0.34, 1.1, 1.2

Quinoa: 0.6, 0.7, 1.1, 1.2, 0.73, 0.59, 0.44, 0.24, 0.85, 0.85

Peanuts: 0.74, 1.3, 0.73, 0.52, 0.26, 0.2, 0.87, 1.1

Oats: 0.62, 1, 1.6, 1.6, 0.82, 0.45, 0.34, 0.29, 1.1, 1

Sesame: 0.85, 0.65, 1.6, 0.88, 0.6, 0.67, 0.45, 1.1, 1

Data compiled by Jen Swallow from US Department of Agriculture, Agricultural Research Service. 2014. USDA National Nutrient Database for Standard Reference, Release 27. Nutrient Data Laboratory home page, http://www.ars.usda.gov/nutrientdata.

Protein and Exercise

The process of building muscle does not have to include supplements.[9, 10] As long as sufficient calories are consumed—and most people eat more than enough food to maintain their weight—there is no need for protein supplements or supplements of any kind in order to build muscle.[9, 10] Even for those engaging in heavy resistance training, supplements are not always necessary for building muscle.[9, 10] However, if calories are restricted or the normal diet is low in protein, then protein supplements may enhance the growth of muscle. In this case, does plant protein stack up against whey protein or meat? Below is a collection of evidence showing that plant protein supplements support muscle growth similar to that of animal protein supplements during resistance training (or in some cases without training).

Plant Protein versus Animal Protein for Muscle Growth

Year	Author	Subjects	Time	Results
2015	Babault et al[11]	161	12 wk	Pea or whey protein groups increased muscle strength/thickness with no difference between groups (50 g/day added protein)
2015	Figueiredo et al[12]	68	16 wk	Soy or whey groups increased muscle mass with no difference between groups (All subjects had Crohn's Disease and were not instructed to exercise, each had 22 g/day added protein)
2013	Joy et al[13]	24	8 wk	Rice or whey increased muscle mass/strength/power with no differences between groups (48 g/day added protein)
2009	Denysschen et al[14]	28	12 wk	Soy, placebo or whey groups increased muscle mass/strength with no difference between groups (26 g/day added protein)
2005	Haub et al[15]	21	14 wk	Soy & beef groups increased strength/muscle power with no difference between groups (0.6 g/kg/day added protein)
2002	Haub et al[16]	21	12 wk	Vegetarian & beef groups increased muscle size/strength with no difference between groups (0.6 g/kg/day added protein)

Protein Can Make You Fat

Many people eat unlimited amounts of protein because they think it does *not* make them fat. I have met with numerous clients, coworkers, and friends who believe that eating more protein cannot possibly result in more body fat. They also believe that there is no limit to how much protein humans should eat, so more is always better. Therefore, the idea of eating more protein and fat through a low-carb diet is appealing to many dieters.

In reality, an excess of *any* type of calories results in weight gain, regardless of whether the calories come from protein or carbs.[17] Three big nutrients known as macronutrients—carbs, fat, and protein—provide calories.[17] Whether reaching excess is more likely on a low-carb or low-fat diet is an area of great controversy.

People often take protein supplements to help them lose weight because they are otherwise cutting total calories. But weight loss is much easier to achieve and maintain in the long-term with a diet based on plant protein instead of meat protein. There are many reasons for this phenomenon. A little-known fact is that plant foods provide fewer calories per gram; they do not fall under the common rule of 4 calories per gram of protein and 9 calories per gram of fat as animal foods do. For example, one gram of protein from beans has 3.47 calories, whereas 1 g of beef protein has 4.27 calories.[1]

Since adults eat close to 100 g of protein each day,[7] this means that plant eaters eat roughly 347 calories for the same amount of protein as meat eaters get for 427 calories. This is an 80-calorie difference for an equal amount of protein between beans and meat. In some cases, such as for artichokes, plant protein is 180 calories lower than animal protein per 100 g.[1] So meat lovers are getting at least 80 calories more than their vegan counterparts eating the same amount of protein every day. This 80-calorie daily difference alone can account for an 8-lb weight gain every year if animal protein is always chosen over plant protein.

This calorie difference is an issue with both protein and fat. Men commonly eat close to 100 g of fat each day,[7] which is equal to 902 calories for animal fat and 837 calories for plant fat. This is a 65-calorie difference, equal to a 6.6-lb weight gain per year. So switching to plant foods can translate to a total weight loss of 14 lb in a year for someone normally getting a combination of fat and protein from animal products. Using oil instead of butter and plant protein instead of meat make significant contributions to weight loss.

Calories per 100 g of Protein and Fat

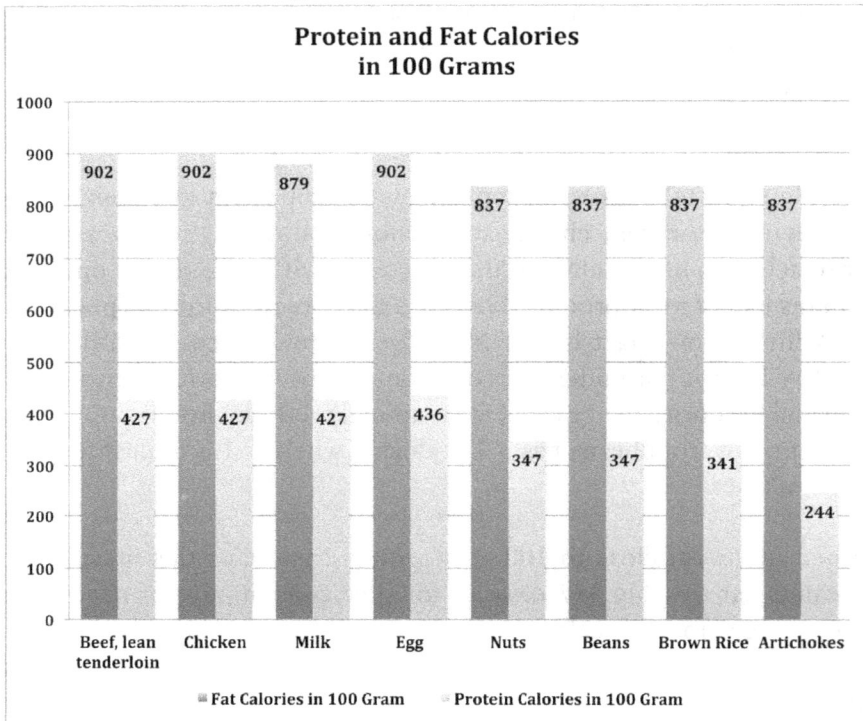

**Protein and Fat Calories
in 100 Grams**

	Beef, lean tenderloin	Chicken	Milk	Egg	Nuts	Beans	Brown Rice	Artichokes
Fat Calories	902	902	879	902	837	837	837	837
Protein Calories	427	427	427	436	347	347	341	244

■ Fat Calories in 100 Gram   Protein Calories in 100 Gram

Data compiled by Jen Swallow from US Department of Agriculture, Agricultural Research Service. 2014. USDA National Nutrient Database for Standard Reference, Release 27. Nutrient Data Laboratory home page, http://www.ars.usda.gov/nutrientdata.

Protein Conclusion

Not only can humans eat enough protein from plant foods, but they can also reap numerous benefits by trading in animal protein for more plant protein. The quality of plant protein is not significantly different or poor when compared with meat protein. There is no need to combine foods at each meal for a balance of amino acids. The protein in foods, such as beans, whole grains, nuts, and seeds, is complete and has enough of the essential amino acids to support building muscle and exercising. In fact, chia seeds stand out as one of the best quality proteins when compared with both animal and other plant foods. Eating these foods can lead to weight loss, which is consistently a major outcome for plant eaters when compared with meat eaters.

In chapters 4 through 7, we established that eating a low-carb diet high in animal protein, such as eggs, dairy, and beef, could indeed contribute to high cholesterol and heart disease. For modern humans trying to live a long and healthy life, these foods should be reduced in order to prevent heart disease, diabetes, and obesity. For these reasons, it is wise to replace at least some animal protein with high-fiber plant protein. Plant protein, after all, works just as well as animal protein.

Notes

1. U.S. Department of Agriculture, Agricultural Research Service. 2014. USDA National Nutrient Database for Standard Reference, Release 27. Nutrient Data Laboratory Home Page, Accessed February 25, 2015, http://www.ars.usda.gov/nutrientdata.
2. Andrich DE, Filion ME, Woods M, Dwyer JT, Gorbach SL, Goldin BR, et al. "Relationship between essential amino acids and muscle mass, independent of habitual diets, in pre- and post-menopausal US women." *Int J Food Sci Nutr* 2011; 62 (7): 719-24.
3. Phillips SM, Moore DR, Tang JE. "A critical examination of dietary protein requirements, benefits, and excesses in athletes." *Int J Sports Nutr Exerc Metab* 2007; 17 Suppl: s58-76.
4. "Nutrition for Everyone, Centers for Disease Control and Prevention", Accessed April, 9 2015, http://www.cdc.gov/nutrition/everyone/basics/protein.html#How%20much%20protein.
5. "Protein, The Nutrition Source, Harvard School of Public Health", Accessed April 9, 2015, http://www.hsph.harvard.edu/nutritionsource/what-should-you-eat/protein/.
6. "Dietary Proteins, Medline Plus, National Institute of Health", Accessed April 9, 2015, http://www.nlm.nih.gov/medlineplus/dietaryproteins.html.

7. "What We Eat in America", NHANES 2011-2012, Accessed April 9, 2015, http://ars.usda.gov/Services/docs.htm?docid=18349.

8. Joint WHO/FAO/UNU Expert Consultation. "Protein and amino acid requirements in human nutrition." *World Health Organ Tech Rep Ser* 2007; (935): 1-265.

9. Herda AA, Herda TJ, Costa PB, Ryan ED, Stout JR, Cramer JT. "Muscle performance, size, and safety responses after eight weeks of resistance training and protein supplementation: a randomized, double-blinded, placebo-controlled clinical trial." *J Strength Cond Res* 2013; 27 (11): 3091-100.

10. Spillane M, Emerson C, Willoughby DS. "The effects of 8 weeks of heavy resistance training and branched-chain amino acid supplementation on body composition and muscle performance." *Nutr Health* 2012; 21 (4): 263-73.

11. Babault N, Paizis C, Deley G, Guerin-Deremaux L, Saniez MH, Lefranc-Millot C, Allaert FA. "Pea proteins oral supplementation promotes muscle thickness gains during resistance training: a double-blind, randomized, placebo-controlled clinical trial vs whey protein." *J Int Soc Sports Nutr* 2015; 12: 3.

12. Figueiredo Machado J, Oya V, Rodrigues Coy CS, Moreno Morcillo A, Dalge Severino S, Wu C, et al. "Whey and soy protein supplements changes body composition in patients with Crohn's Disease undergoing Azathioprine and anti-TNF-alpha therapy." *Nutr Hosp* 2015; 31 (n04): 1603-1610.

13. Joy JM, Lowery RP, Wilson JM, Purpura M, De Souza EO, Wilson SM, et al. "The effects of 8 weeks of whey or rice protein supplementation on body composition and exercise performance." *Nutr* 2013; 12: 86.

14. Denyschen CA, Burton HW, Horvath PJ, Leddy JJ, Browne RW. "Resistance training with soy vs whey protein supplements in hyperlipidemic males." *J Int Soc Sports Nutr* 2009; 6: 8.

15. Haub MD, Wells AM, Campbell WW. "Beef and soy-based food supplements differentially affect cerum lipoprotein lipid profiles because of changes in carbohydrate intake and novel nutrient intake ratios in older men who resistive-train." *Metabolism* 2005; 54 (6): 769-74.

16. Haub MD, Wells AM, Tarnopolsky MA, Campbell WW. "Effect of protein source on resistive-training-induced changes in body composition and muscle size in older men." *Am J Clin Nutr* 2002; 76 (3): 511-7.

17. "Finding a Balance", Centers for Disease Control and Prevention, Accessed February 19, 2015, http://www.cdc.gov/healthyweight/calories/.

18. Bowman SA, Spence JT. "A comparison of low-carbohydrate vs. high carbohydrate diets: energy restriction, nutrient quality and correlation to body mass index." *J Am Coll Nutr* 2002; 21 (3): 268-74.

19. Kennedy ET, Bowman SA, Spence JT, Freedman M, King J. "Popular diets: correlation to health, nutrition, and obesity." *J Am Diet Assoc* 2001; 101 (4): 411-20.

20. Macdiarmid JI, Cade JE, Blundell JE. "High and low fat consumers, their macronutrient intake and body mass index: further analysis of the National Diet and Nutrition Survey of British Adults." *Eur J Clin Nutr* 1996; 50 (8): 505-12.

21. Bradbury KE, Crowe FL, Appleby PN, Schmidt JA, Travis RC, Key TJ. "Serum concentrations of cholesterol, apolipoprotein A-1 and apolipoprotein B in a total of 1694 meat-eaters, fish-eaters, vegetarians and vegans." *Eur J Clin Nutr* 2014; 68 (2): 178-83.

22. Tonstad SI, Stewart K, Oda K, Batech M, Herring RP, Fraser GE. "Vegetarian diets and incidence of diabetes in the Adventist Health Study-2." *Nutr Metab Cardiovasc* 2013; 23 (4): 292-9.

23. Gilsing AMJ, Crowe FL, Lloyd-Wright Z, Sanders TAB, Appleby PN, Allen NE, Key TJ. "Serum concentrations of vitamin B12 and folate in British male omnivores, vegetarians and vegans: results from a cross-sectional analysis of the EPIC-Oxford cohort study." *Eur J Clin Nutr* 2010; 64 (9): 933-939.

24. Robinson-O'Brien R, Perry CL, Wall MM, Story M, Neumark-Sztainer D. "Adolescent and young adults vegetarianism: better dietary intake and weight outcomes but increased risk of disordered eating behaviors." *J Am Diet Assoc* 2009; 109 (4): 648-655.

25. Tonstad S, Butler T, Yan R, Fraser GE. "Types of vegetarian diet, body weight, and prevalence of type 2 diabetes." *Diabetes Care* 2009; 32 (5): 791-6.

26. Rosell M, Appleby P, Spencer E, Key T. "Weight gain over 5 years in 21,966 meat-eating, fish-eating, vegetarian, and vegan men and women in EPIC-Oxford." *Int J Obes* 2006; 30: 1389-1396.

27. Newby PK, Tucker KL, Wolk A. "Risk of overweight and obesity among semivegetarian, lactovegetarian, and vegan women." *Am J Clin Nutr* 2005; 81 (6): 1267-74.

28. Spencer EA Int, Appleby PN, Davey GK, Key TJ. "Diet and body mass index in 38000 EPIC-Oxford meat-eaters, fish-eaters, vegetarians and vegans." *Int J Obes Relat Metab Disord* 2003; 27 (6): 728-34.

29. Janelle KC, Barr SI. "Nutrient intakes and eating behavior scores of vegetarian and nonvegetarian women." *J Am Diet Assoc* 1995; 95 (2): 180-6.

CHAPTER 8

To Gluten or Not to Gluten?

Claims that gluten causes inflammation and weight gain have driven multitudes to go gluten-free. The Paleo diet is gluten-free and allegedly lowers inflammation, thereby combating autoimmune diseases and obesity.[1,2] But where is the evidence for this claim, and is it really the Paleo diet or just the effects of weight loss that impact inflammation?

What is inflammation? If you have ever bumped your head really hard and it started swelling a few hours later, then you have experienced a process in the body called inflammation. This kind of reaction is temporary (or acute, as clinicians call it). Inflammation accompanied by redness, heat, and swelling is what normally happens during injury or illness.[3,4] The body reacts in a similar fashion to viruses or injury with a release of proinflammatory proteins called cytokines to help repair damaged tissue.[3] Another kind of inflammation, which is not acute or temporary, is called chronic inflammation because it can last for years instead of just a few days or weeks.

A common way that doctors can measure how much chronic inflammation is in the body is by taking blood and testing it for a protein called high sensitivity C-reactive protein (hs CRP). Release of proinflammatory cytokines can be a good thing if it is just temporary until the injury is healed. On the other hand, inflammation that is high or even mildly high for long periods of time is dangerous. This chronic inflammation is associated with chronic illnesses like heart disease, type 2 diabetes, dementia,[5] metabolic syndrome,[6] and Alzheimer's disease.[3]

Gluten and Inflammation

Does gluten cause inflammation in the general population? How common is this problem? A small fraction of the population has wheat allergies or celiac disease, which means they cannot tolerate wheat or gluten. The most common food allergies, including wheat allergies, affect about 3% of the population.[7, 8] When individuals with wheat allergies consume wheat, they experience a reaction that involves inflammation.[9]

Young children with wheat allergies often outgrow these allergies.[8–11] Common reactions from wheat allergies are vomiting, diarrhea, low blood pressure, and skin rashes.[8] In this case, a test called immunoglobulin E or IgE antibody is used to confirm this allergy.[11]

Celiac disease is an autoimmune digestive disease that damages the small intestine and interferes with the absorption of nutrients.[12] Indeed, patients with celiac disease experience inflammation upon digesting wheat or gluten.[13] Patients with this disease also commonly experience weight loss, anemia, vomiting, and diarrhea when they consume gluten or foods with gluten residue.[12] Think you might have this disease? Celiac disease is rare in Caucasians as it only affects about 1% of the population.[14] It is even less common in minority groups, such as Hispanic or African American populations.[14]

Gluten Sensitivity

Is it possible to have a reaction to wheat if you do not have a wheat allergy or celiac disease? A relatively new diagnosis called nonceliac gluten sensitivity (NCGS) was developed to describe patients reacting to wheat reporting digestive and nondigestive symptoms.[15] NCGS patients test negative for celiac and wheat allergies.[15] Scientists may identify NCGS with a variety of targeted immune tests.[15]

So it is possible to react to wheat without an allergy or celiac disease. If you experience hives, vomiting, or diarrhea immediately or soon after eating gluten, you may want to avoid eating it. But the question of whether wheat intake in the general population causes chronic inflammation leading to heart disease, diabetes, or other deadly chronic diseases remains.

To answer this question, we can look at the relationship between inflammatory biomarkers and wheat/gluten intake. For example, researchers at the University of Eastern Finland found that eating a whole-grain-enriched diet was associated with a *decrease* in hs CRP levels, one marker of inflammation.[16] Other markers of inflammation, such as TNF-α, IL-1β, and IL-6, *decreased* in another study in which patients increased wheat intake, regardless of whether it was whole grain.[17] In special populations, such as diabetic women, whole-grain intake is still linked to *lower* inflammation, whereas refined grains may increase inflammation.[18]

Keep in mind that both whole grains and refined grains contain gluten. If one lowers inflammation while the other does not, then something besides the gluten is responsible for this phenomenon. The fact that whole grains have more fiber and magnesium[20] may be why they can lower inflammation.[19, 21]

Reviewing the relationship—*if* there is one between wheat intake and heart disease, obesity, or diabetes—might also help us understand the consequences of eating wheat. If wheat, gluten, and grains in general were the cause of inflammation, then eating them would increase the risk of heart disease, diabetes, and other inflammation-related diseases. An overwhelming amount of evidence points to the contrary.[22–26] Whole-grain intake can reduce the risk of heart disease by up to 40% when habitual whole-grain eaters are compared with those who eat them rarely.[22] Eating three servings of whole grains per day can reduce the risk of type 2 diabetes by up to 30%.[26]

Overall, eating whole grains may independently lower all-cause mortality.[23] Scientific evidence, therefore, indicates that gluten intake, as long as it is only consumed in the form of whole grains, lowers inflammation.[23] This is because it lowers the risk of diseases such as heart disease, diabetes, and possibly even cancer.[23] This is likely due to the soluble fiber content of whole grains, but may also be due to phytoestrogens and antioxidants. Aside from the fiber and vitamin content of whole grains, there may be additional reasons why they are able to help lower the risk of chronic diseases, such as their effects on gut bacteria.[27]

What Causes Inflammation?

If grains and gluten do not cause inflammation, then what does? Obese and elderly people tend to have detectable levels of inflammation throughout the body called low-grade systemic inflammation.[28, 29] This phenomenon is directly influenced by weight: if weight decreases, so does inflammation.[29-32] Body fat, particularly belly fat, is linked to low-grade systemic inflammation, which becomes chronic because it remains high long-term.[32]

What far-reaching consequences does this discovery have? Think of how many people are suffering from low-grade inflammation: most adults in the United States are overweight or obese.[33] This means that nearly 70% of American adults are living with this inflammation that is associated with heart disease, cancer, diabetes, and more.

More Inflammation

So how do we stop this terrible epidemic from ruining our health? Paleo advocates claim that their diet is great for lowering this kind of low-grade inflammation. In reality, anything that helps people lose weight can temporarily lower inflammation.[29-32]

Is it really that simple, that less body fat equals less inflammation? Not exactly, as other things cause inflammation besides body fat. Eating fat triggers body fat to produce inflammation.[34] That's right: Dietary fat may be more of a villain than carbs. But not just any fat; specifically, saturated fat intake leads to inflammation.[33-37] This is one explanation why the typical

American diet loaded with high-fat foods like pizza, hamburgers, hot dogs, sausage, cake, and donuts creates a proinflammatory state in the body.[35, 36]

What other foods cause inflammation? University of Leicester Professor Clett Erridge analyzed twenty-seven common foods in the Western diet by testing extracts of these foods in vitro with human cells.[38] Bread (which contains gluten), chips, veggies, fruits, pork, turkey, yogurt, and many more foods were included in these experiments. Only a few of these foods induced a significant inflammatory response from human cells, and gluten-containing bread was not one of them.[38]

Turkey, pork, cheese, yogurt, chocolate, and ice cream were the top proinflammatory culprits in these experiments.[38] The bacteria that grows on these foods seems to influence how much inflammation they cause, but cooking them does not solve the problem. In fact, even after cooking meat for an hour, it still retains a significant amount of proinflammatory activity.[39] The question remains: Does this series of experiments with human cells in petri dishes translate to real life?

Yes, in fact; beef consumption for several weeks can raise CRP significantly in healthy men[40] and women.[41] Researchers at the University of Navarra in Spain put ninety-six people on an experimental low-carb diet and a control diet.[42] Even though both groups lost weight, the group who ate more animal protein and meat had higher inflammation than those who ate more vegetable protein or fish.[42] Vegetable protein sources include grains, beans, nuts, and seeds. The type of dietary protein is, therefore, more important than the amount for affecting inflammation, despite the fact that weight loss itself lowers inflammation.

If the experiments described earlier with proinflammatory foods could be applied to real life, then permanently cutting out foods like meat and dairy could lower inflammation in the human body. Indeed, a vegetarian diet counteracts inflammatory diseases.[43] Some of this may be due to the fact that vegetarians are usually leaner than omnivores. But if the vegetarian diet can protect against obesity, then why not take advantage of this benefit as well? Furthermore, one month of eating a vegan diet, which excludes all dairy, egg, and meat/poultry, can significantly lower inflammation.[44] Just twenty-one days of eating a whole-food diet free of animal products can lower CRP by 40% along with reducing cholesterol and triglycerides.[45]

Looking at people who had a meatless diet for years and comparing them to meat eaters offers practical insights on disease rates. When healthy meat eaters are compared with vegetarians, the vegetarian diet is associated with lower inflammation in American,[44] Asian,[46] and Slovakian studies.[47] This supports the data from short-term experimental studies on inflammation and diet. Of course, committing to a healthy plant-based diet long-term is even better than just trying it for a month.

Less Inflammation

What about legumes? Beans, lentils, and peas are part of a food group called legumes, which are bad guys in the Paleo world. Caveman diet proponents claim that legumes were not a natural food for prehistoric man and contain dangerous toxins known as lectins.[48] These toxins supposedly damage the walls of the intestines and contribute to several unwanted side effects, such as leaky gut, weight gain, headaches, and depression.[48] A leaky gut is said to cause autoimmune diseases such as thyroiditis, Crohn's disease, celiac disease, and rheumatoid arthritis. These diseases are generally associated with inflammation. But do beans increase inflammation?

Raw dried beans do contain a significant amount of lectins and substances that lower mineral absorption, such as phytates.[49] Phytates are known as antinutrients because they can decrease the absorption of some minerals.[50] They do not steal minerals from the body or leach minerals from bones. For example, normal levels of phytates in grains and legumes can decrease the digestibility of protein up to 10%.[50] This means that you may absorb 13.5 of the 15 g of protein found in one cup of kidney beans. Phytates are found in raw and cooked beans, but lectins are reduced in canned and cooked beans.[52, 53] The canning process also increases protein digestibility.[53] So when was the last time you had the urge to rip open a bag of raw dried pinto beans and pop them into your mouth like a handful of potato chips? Probably never.

Most people typically cook their food, especially meat and beans. Raw meat has its disadvantages, such as E. coli or other food-borne illness-causing bacteria, but some people continue to eat raw meat and sashimi. The same goes for eating raw eggs and salmonella poisoning. Eating raw dried beans would be more like eating a very hard, immature, unripe fruit. Not only does it taste bad, it is not ready for consumption. All food should be harvested at the right time or prepared properly in order to avoid illness or unwanted side effects.

Soaking overnight not only makes dry beans easier to digest, but it also increases their antioxidant activity.[49, 51] Think of how seeds sprout and grow after adequate rainfall. In a wild setting, immature beans would eventually be exposed to rain or moisture and germinate. This is the stage that makes them easier to digest. Boiling beans after soaking and germinating them can diminish lectins among other antinutritional factors.[52, 53] The point is that beans and whole grains are not the enemy. As long as these foods are prepared or cooked properly, they are a healthy alternative to bacon or steak. Eating more of these foods can increase fiber intake and lower cholesterol. Bacon and steak have plenty of fat but no fiber.

There are many reasons why vegetarians tend to have lower inflammation. Just as there are proinflammatory foods, there are also anti-inflammatory foods, most of which include plants. Though legumes, also known as beans, are a Paleo no-no, they have proven to be a key player in good health. One reason for this is that beans, such as garbanzo and kidney beans, have an anti-inflammatory effect.[54] According to one study, eating merely four servings of legumes per week can lower serum CRP levels by 40% in two months.[54]

If beans are the princes, then nuts are the kings of the anti-inflammatory realm. In addition to a healthy diet, increasing nut consumption by 1.4 g, which is the equivalent of one almond or half a walnut per day, is associated with a 49% decrease in mortality from chronic inflammatory diseases.[55] Other foods proven to lower inflammation are extra virgin olive oil, tomato juice, red wine, flaxseed meal, black tea, and sweet cherries.[56, 57]

Whole fruits are commonly accepted as a health food with fiber, vitamin, antioxidants, and practically no fat. Fruit juices are often under attack because of the amount of sugar they contain, but there is a big difference between drinking 100% orange juice and drinking an orange soda, or worse, an artificial orange-flavored energy drink. At least juice has some natural vitamins and minerals, such as vitamin C and potassium, without the added caffeine or phosphoric acid found in soda.

I would not recommend having more than a cup of juice each day, especially for weight-loss purposes, because of the high number of calories per serving. The only exception to that rule is making fresh vegetable juice combined with fruit in a juicer. This would be better than buying bottled and pasteurized juice. Vitamins are light and heat sensitive, so they are damaged somewhat during processing and over time. In addition to other advantages, eating vegetables can be beneficial due to their anti-inflammatory effect.[56, 57]

Making a fresh veggie juice can ensure that more nutrients are unharmed. Though no more than a cup should be consumed each day, fruit juice appears to have some benefits that people are unaware of. For example, drinking a cup of pomegranate juice each day can lower inflammatory markers in the blood.[58]

Fruits, vegetables, beans, and nuts can be like an army protecting the body against inflammation when they are included in the diet regularly. Excess saturated fat appears to be a villain that threatens that army. What about unsaturated fat? Does it have the same effects? It depends on which fats we are talking about. Some unsaturated fats have anti-inflammatory effects as opposed to saturated fats, which can cause inflammation.[59, 60]

Not only do Americans eat too much saturated fat, but they also consume too much omega-6 unsaturated fats.[59] The ratio of omega-6 to omega-3 fats is important for good health. Vegetable oil, salad dressing, fried foods, and mayo are high in omega-6, while walnuts, flaxseeds, chia seeds, and fish are high in omega-3. An omega-6 to omega-3 ratio of 2 to 1 or even 3 to 1 is better to prevent diseases than the current ratio Americans eat, which can be as high as 15 to 1.[59] Omega-3 intake is associated with lower levels of inflammation.[59] Eating more omega-3 is not enough; the amount of omega-6 needs to go down at the same time to really make a difference.[59]

Gluten Conclusion

The bottom line is that Americans should focus more on a permanent and healthy solution to weight loss without the emphasis on gluten-free foods. Weight loss, *no matter how you achieve it*, has a major effect on inflammation.[63] Obese people who eat gluten, or low-carb or low-fat diets, can all lower their inflammation by losing a significant amount of body fat.[57] Plant-based diets, however, have the advantage when it comes to keeping inflammation down once weight is stable.[43–47] One way this works is by using beans and nuts as protein sources, which can drastically affect inflammation.[48, 49]

The fate of inflammation is much more about weight and overall diet than it is about gluten. Additionally, as people eat more whole grains and beans, the body adapts to phytate intake and is able to absorb more minerals, such as iron, from these foods.[64] This is a beneficial effect especially for women with low iron stores.[64] For these reasons, Americans can benefit from trading all of their white/refined grain foods for whole-grain foods.[23]

Notes

1. "Paleo Diet, Inflammation and Metformin", Robb Wolf, Accessed March 18, 2015, http://robbwolf.com/2012/03/09/paleo-diet-inflammation-metformin/.
2. "The Paleo Diet and the Gluten Free Lifestyle", Becky Rider, Accessed March 18, 2015, http://www.living-gluten-free.com/paleo.html.

3. Giunta B, Fernandez F, Nikolic W, et al. "Inflammaging as a prodome to Alzheimer's disease." *J Neuroinflammation* 2008; 5: 51.

4. Cinat ME, Waxman K, Granger GA, Pearce W, et al. "Trauma causes sustained elevation of soluble tumor necrosis factor receptors." *J Am Coll Surg* 1994; 179 (5): 529-37.

5. Bartlett DB, Firth CM, Phillips AC, et al. "The age-related increase in low-grade systemic inflammation (inflammaging) is not driven by cytomegalovirus infection." *Aging Cell* 2012; 11 (5): 912-15.

6. Abdullah AR, Hasan HA, Raiganger VL. "Analysis of the relationship of leptin, high-sensitivity C-reactive protein, adiponectin, insulin, and uric acid to metabolic syndrome in lean, overweight, and obese young females." *Metab Syndr Relat Disord* 2009; 7 (1): 17-22.

7. Vierk KA, Koehler KM, Fein SB, Street DA. "Prevalence of self-reported food allergy in American adults and use of food labels." *J Allergy Clin Immunol* 2007; 119 (6): 1504-10.

8. Nowak-Wegrzyn A, Conover-Walker MK, Wood RA. "Food-allergic reactions in schools and preschools." *Arch Pediatr Adolesc Med* 2001; 155 (7): 790-5.

9. Valenta R, Hochwallner H, Linhart B, Pahr S. "Food allergies-the basics." *Gastroenterology* 2015. [Epub ahead of print.]

10. Eller E, Kjaer HF, Host A, Andersen KE, Bindslev-Jensen C. "Food allergy and food sensitization in early childhood: results from the DARC cohort." *Allergy* 2009; 64 (7): 1023-9.

11. Ostblom E, Lilja G, Pershagen G, van Hage M, Wickman M. "Phenotypes of food hypersensitivity and development of allergic diseases during the first 8 years of life." *Clin Exp Allergy* 2008; 38 (8): 1325-32.

12. "Celiac Disease", US Dept of Health and Human Services, National Institute of Diabetes and Digestive Diseases, Accessed March 18, 2015, http://www.niddk.nih.gov/health-information/health-topics/digestive-diseases/celiac-disease/Pages/facts.aspx.

13. Silano M, Pozo EP, Uberti F, Manferdelli S, Del Pinto T, Felli C, et al. "Diversity of oat varieties in eliciting the early inflammatory events in celiac disease." *Eur J Nutr* 2014; 53 (5): 1177-86.

14. Rubio-Tapia A, Ludvigsson JF, Brantner TL, Murray JA, Everhart JE. "The prevalence of celiac disease in the United States." *Am J Gastroenterol* 2012; 107 (10): 1538-44.

15. Mansueto P, Seidita A, D'Alcamo A, Carroccio A. "Non-celiac gluten sensitivity : literature review." *J Am Coll Nutr* 2014; 33 (1): 39-54.

16. De Mello VD, Schwab U, Kolehmainen M, Koenig W, Siloaho M, Poutanen K, et al. "A diet high in fatty fish, bilberries and wholegrain products improves markers of endothelial function and inflammation in individuals with impaired glucose metabolism in a randomised controlled trial : the Sysdimet study." *Diabetologia* 2011; 54 (11): 2755-67.

17. Langkamp-Henken B, Nieves C Jr, Culpepper T, Radford A, Girard SA, Hughes C, et al. "Fecal lactic acid bacteria increased in adolescents randomized to whole-grain but not refined-grain foods, whereas inflammatory cytokine production decreased equally with both interventions. " *J Nutr* 2012; 142 (11): 2025-32.

18. Qi L, van Dam RM, Liu S, Franz M, Mantzoros C, Hu FB. "Whole-grain, bran, and cereal fiber intakes and markers of systemic inflammation in diabetic women." *Diabetes Care* 2006; 29 (2): 207-11.

19. Ma Y, Hebert JR, Li W, Bertone-Johnson ER, Olendzki B, Pagoto SL, et al. "Association between dietary fiber and markers of systemic inflammation in the Women's Health Initiative Observational Study." *Nutrition* 2008; 24 (10): 941-9.

20. U.S. Department of Agriculture, Agricultural Research Service. 2014. USDA National Nutrient Database for Standard Reference, Release 27. Nutrient Data Laboratory Home Page, Accessed February 25, 2015, http://www.ars.usda.gov/nutrientdata.

21. Song Y, Li TY, van Dam RM, Manson JE, Hu FB. "Magnesium intake and plasma concentrations of markers of systemic inflammation and endothelial dysfunction in women." *Am J Clin Nutr* 2007; 85 (4): 1068-74.

22. Flight I, Clifton P. "Cereal grains and legumes in the prevention of coronary heart disease and stroke : a review of the literature." *Eur J Clin Nutr* 2006 ;60(10) :1145-59.

23. Wu H, Flint AJ, Qi Q, van Dam RM, Simpson LA, Rimm EB, et al. "Association between dietary whole grain intake and risk of mortality : two large prospective studies in US men and women." *JAMA Intern Med* 2015 ;175(3) :373-84.

24. Wu Y, Qian Y, Pan Y, Li P, Yang J, Ye X, Xu G. "Association between dietary fiber intake and risk of coronary heart disease : A meta-analysis." *Clin Nutr* 2014. [Epub ahead of print]

25. Kim Y, Je Y. Dietary fiber intake and total mortality : a meta-analysis of prospective cohort studies." *Am J Epidemiol* 2014 ;180(6) :565-73.

26. Venn BJ, Mann JI. "Cereal grains, legumes and diabetes." *Eur J Clin Nutr* 2004; 58 (11): 1443-61.

27. Ross AB, Pere-Trepat E, Montoliu I, Martin FP, Collino S, Moco S, et al. "A whole-grain-rich diet reduces urinary excretion of markers of protein catabolism and gut microbiota metabolism in healthy men after one week." *J Nutr* 2013; 143 (6): 766-73.

28. Kahn SE, Zinman B, Haffner SM, et al. "Obesity is a major determinant of the association of C-reactive protein levels and the metabolic syndrome in type 2 diabetes." *Diabetes* 2006; 55 (8): 2357-64.

29. Catalan V, Gomez-Ambrosi J, Rodriguez A, Ramirez B, Rotellar F, Valenti V, Silva C, Gil MJ, Fernandez-Real JM, Salvador J, Fruhbeck G. "Increased levels of calprotectin in obesity are related to macrophage content: impact on inflammation and effect of weight loss." *Mol Med* 2011; 17: (11-12): 1157–1167.

30. Esposito K, Pontillo A, Ciotola M, Di Palo C, Grella E, Nicoletti G, Guiglano D. "Weight loss reduces interleukin-18 levels in obese women." *J Clin Endocrinol Metab* 2002; 87: 3864-3866.

31. Ziccardi P, Nappo F, Guiglano G, Esposito K, Marfella R, Cioffi M, D'Andrea F, Molinari AM, Guiglano D. "Reduction of inflammatory cytokine concentrations and improvement of endothelial functions in obese women after weight loss over one year." *Circulation* 2002; 105: 804-809.

32. Park JS, Cho MH, Nam JS, et al. "Visceral adiposity and leptin are independently associated with C-reactive protein in Korean type 2 diabetic patients." *Acta Diabetol* 2010; 47 (2): 113-8.

33. Flegal KM, Carroll MD, Ogden CL, Curtin LR. "Prevalence and trends in obesity among US adults, 1999-2008." *JAMA* 2010, 303; 235-241.

34. Van Dijk SJ, Feskens JM, Bos MB, Hoelen DWM, Heijligenberg R, Bromhaar MG, de Groot L, de Vries JHM, Muller M, Afman LA. "A saturated fatty acid-rich diet induces an obesity-linked proinflammatory gene expression profile in adipose tissue of subjects at risk of metabolic syndrome." *Am J Clin Nutr* 2009; 90: 6: 1656-1664.

35. Burdge GC, PC Calder. "Plasma cytokine response during the postprandial period: a potential causal process in vascular disease?" *Brit J Nutr* 2005; 93: 3-9.

36. Seaman DR. "The diet-induced proinflammatory state: a cause of chronic pain and other degenerative diseases?" *J Manipul Physiol Therap.* 2002; 25: 3: 168-179.

37. Nappo F, Esposito K, Cioffi M, Guigliano G, Molinari AM, Paolisso G, Marfella R, Guigliano D. "Postprandial endothilial activation in healthy subjects and in type 2 diabetic patients: role of fat and carbohydrate meals." *J Am Coll Cardiol.* 2002; 39: 1145-1150.

38. Erridge C. "The capacity of foodstuffs to induce innate immune activation of human monocytes in vitro is dependent on food content of stimulants of Toll-like receptors 2 and 4." *Brit J Nutr* 2011; 105: 15-23.

39. Erridge C. "Accumulation of stimulants of Toll-like receptor (TLR)-2 and TLR4 in meat products stored at 5° C." *J Food Sci* 2011; 76 (2): H72-9.

40. McDaniel J, Askew W, Bennett D, et al. "Bison meat has a lower atherogenic risk than beef in healthy men." *Nutr Res* 2013; 33 (4): 293-302.

41. Ley SH, Sun Q, Willett WC, Eliassen AH, Wu K, Pan A, et al. "Associations between red meat intake and biomarkers of inflammation and glucose metabolism in women." *Am J Clin Nutr* 2014; 99 (2): 352-60.

42. Lopez-Legarrea P, de la Iglesia R, Abete I, et al. "The protein type within a hypocaloric diet affects obesity-related inflammation: the RESMENA project." *Nutr* 2014; 30 (4): 424-9.

43. Paalani M, Lee JW, Haddad E, Tonstad S. "Determinants of inflammatory markers in a bi-ethnic population." *Ethn Dis* 2011; 21 (2): 142-9.

44. Kim MS, Hwang SS, Park EJ, Bae JW. "Strict vegetarian diet improves the risk factors associated with metabolic diseases by modulating gut microbiota and reducing intestinal inflammation." *Environ Microbiol Rep* 2013; 5 (5): 765-75.

45. Alleman RJ, Harvey IC, Farney TM, Bloomer RJ. "Both a traditional and modified Daniel Fast improve the cardio-metabolic profile in men and women." *Lipids Health Dis 2013*; 12 (1): 114.

46. Chen CW, Lin YL, Lin TK, Lin CT, et al. "Total cardiovascular risk profile of Taiwanese vegetarians." *Eur J Clin Nutr* 2008; 62 (1): 138-44.

47. Krajcovicova-Kudlackova M, Blazicek P. "C-reactive protein and nutrition." *Bratisl Lek Listy* 2005; 106 (11): 345-7.

48. "Why No Grains and Legumes? Part 1: Lectins", Accessed September 5, 2015, http://www.paleoplan.com/2011/03-30/why-no-grains-and-legumes/.

49. Aguilera Y, Diaz MF, Jimenez T, Benitez V, Herrera T, Cuadrado C, et al. "Changes in nonnutritional factors and antioxidant activity during germination of legumes." *J Agric Food Chem* 2013; 61 (34): 8120-5.

50. Sarwar Gilani G, Wu Xiao C, Cockell KA. "Impact of antinutritional factors in food proteins on the digestibility of protein and the bioavailability of amino acids and on protein quality." *Br J Nutr* 2012; 108 Suppl 2: s315-32.

51. Chon Su. "Total polyphenols and bioactivity of seeds and sprouts in several legumes." *Curr Pharm Des* 2013; 19 (34): 6112-24.

52. Sotelo A, Argote RM, Moreno RI, Flores NI, Diaz M. "Nutritive evaluation of the seed, germinated seed, and string bean of Erythrina Americana and the detoxification of the material by boiling." *J Agric Food Chem* 2003; 51 (9): 2821-5.

53. Savelkoul FH, van der Poel AF, Tamminga S. "The presence and activation of trypsin inhibitors, tannins, lectins and amylase inhibitors in legume seeds during germination. A review." *Plant Foods Hum Nutr* 1992; 42 (1): 71-85.

54. Hermsdorff HHM, Zulet MA, Abete I, Martinez JA. "A legume-based hypocaloric diet reduces pro-inflammatory status and improves metabolic features in overweight/obese subjects." *Eur J Nutr* 2011; 50: 61-69.

55. Gopinath B, Buyken AE, Flood VM, Empsom M, Rochtchina E, Mitchell P. "Consumption of polyunsaturated fatty acids, fish, and nuts and risk of inflammatory disease mortality." *Am J Clin Nutr* 2011; 93 (5): 1073-9.

56. Watzl B. "Anti-inflammatory effects of plant-based foods and of their constituents." *Int J Vitam Nutr Res* 2008; 78 (6): 293-8.

57. Nettleton JA, Steffen LM, Mayer-Davis EJ, et al. "Dietary patterns are associated with biochemical markers of inflammation and endothelial activation in the Multi-ethnic study of atherosclerosis (MESA)." *Am J Clin Nutr* 2006; 83 (6): 1369-79.

58. Sohrab G, Nasrollahzadeh J, Zand H. "Effects of pomegranate juice consumption on inflammatory markers in patients with type 2 diabetes: A randomized, placebo controlled study." *J Res Med Sci* 2014;19 (3): 215-220.

59. Simopoulos AP. "The importance of the ratio of omega-6/omega-3 essential fatty acids." *Biomed Pharmacother* 2002, 56 (8): 365-79.

60. Murakami K, Sasaki S, Takahashi Y, et al. "Total n-3 polyunsaturated fatty acid intake is inversely associated with serum C-reactive protein in young Japanese women." *Nutr Res* 2008; 28 (5): 309-14.

61. Niu K, Hozawa A, Kuriyama S, et al. "Dietary long-chain n-3 fatty acids of marine origin and serum C-reactive protein concentrations are associated in a population with a diet rich in marine products." *Am J Clin Nutr* 2006; 84 (1): 223-9.

62. Hoyos C, Almqvist C, Garden F, et al. "Effect of omega 3 and omega 6 fatty acid intakes from diet and supplements on plasma fatty acid levels in the first 3 years of life." *Asia Pac J Clin Nutr* 2008; 17 (4): 552-7.

63. Nicklas JM, Sacks FM, Smith SR, LeBoff MS, Rood JC, Bray GA, et al. "Effect of dietary composition of weight loss diets on high-sensitivity c-reactive protein: the Randomized POUNDS LOST trial." *Obesity (Silver Spring)* 2013; 21 (4): 681-9.

64. Armah SM, Boy E, Chen D, Candal P, Reddy MB. "Regular consumption of a high phytate diet reduces the inhibitory effect of phytate on nonheme-iron absorption in women with suboptimal iron stores." *Am Soc Nutr* 2015; 145 (8): 1735-9.

CHAPTER 9

Inflammation, Aging, and Meat

What if you just eat a low-fat and high-protein diet with moderate amounts of lean meat? That way you could enjoy at least a small serving of lean meat at each meal, right? This idea is probably what draws so many people to the Paleo diet. A little steak or BBQ chicken sounds so much more appetizing than a bowl of beans to many people at first. Eating lean meat with plenty of veggies seems healthy from a perspective of simply looking at how much fat, protein, or carbs we eat and how to minimize processed foods.

Which diet is best for overall health? As I hope you are beginning to realize, Paleo, or low-carb dieting in general, is not the healthiest choice according to all the data presented in this book. Paleo followers can lose weight in the first few months of dieting. A high intake of animal products, however, is likely to make them regain the weight as time goes on.[1-4] The temporary weight loss can lead to temporary drops in blood pressure and cholesterol, but as the weight is regained, those numbers can also increase. Each increase of 250 g per day in chicken, red meat, or processed meat can account for a weight gain of about a pound per year.[3] This translates to a large steak, half a large chicken breast, or two burger patties. On the Paleo diet, total meat intake easily adds up to well over 500 g. If breakfast includes a serving of bacon, lunch is a steak and veggies, and dinner is an equivalent sized piece of chicken with veggies, then meat intake would be over 500 g.

The main reason why some Paleo dieters experience quick weight loss is due to the removal of unhealthy processed foods like cookies, donuts, cheese, fries, candy, and soda. Processed foods are easy to overeat, while whole foods are more filling per calorie. A diet of processed foods is usually higher in calories when compared with a whole-food diet. A whole-food diet can be simple, nutritious, and enjoyable, but any diet can be difficult at times because we all have cravings and momentary urges to eat something tasty. These cravings rarely point us in the direction of produce. Calorie restrictions and general compliance, no matter what type of diet is involved, becomes increasingly difficult after a few months of dieting.

Weight loss should not be the only factor considered when choosing a diet. Many reasons exist, besides saturated fat and cholesterol, why foregoing legumes and grains for more meat can be harmful and why the low-carb diet can be deadly.[5-13] In the long-term, these kinds of diets actually raise the risks of cancer, heart disease, diabetes, and all-cause mortality.[5-13] This scenario can be worse for those who already have a chronic disease.[7]

How Much Meat Is Considered Healthy?

We saw how fat and cholesterol intake might affect the risk of heart disease for diabetics. For those who try to reduce fat intake on the Paleo diet, this diet is still high in cholesterol, which means it can hurt people who already have diabetes. Furthermore, this kind of diet can be more harmful for those diagnosed with heart disease.[7] Eating less protein, closer to 10% of total calories from protein, on the other hand, may lower the risk of these diseases in contrast to the trendy caveman diet, which is more than double the protein.[10-12]

Another problem with the Paleo mindset is that saturated fat and cholesterol are not the only harmful substances we can get from indulging in meat. Every protein food—whether it is fish, chicken, peanut butter, tofu, beans, or whole grains—has some benefits and some downsides. Regardless of whether the food is 100% natural or pure, there are pros and cons to each choice. The taste of steak is more appetizing to many people than the taste of beans, so this is a pro for steak, but the lack of fiber is a con.

Where you get your protein is just as or even more important than *how much* protein you eat. Lean meat is more than just a source of protein. In addition to antibiotic residues and heavy metals, lean meat contains some substances that are harmful when consumed in excess, including:

- AGEs
- Heme iron
- Dietary carcinogens

AGEs

Perhaps the most harmful compounds in meat are advanced glycation end products (AGEs), which are a group of substances that form due to reactions between certain sugars and proteins, fats, or nucleic acids.[14–18] Some amount of AGEs, also known as glycotoxins, already exist naturally in the human body and in raw foods, but the body can absorb more from dietary intake.[17] AGEs accumulate and cause widespread damage to cells and organs in the body via increased oxidant stress and inflammation.[18–20] When high levels accumulate in tissue and circulation, they become pathogenic. This kind of stress and inflammation is linked to many diseases, such as diabetes and cardiovascular disease, in addition to accelerated aging.[17]

Cooking foods, especially with dry heat, increases the formation of AGEs by tenfold to a hundredfold. High-temperature cooking like grilling, broiling, searing, frying, and roasting results in the highest amounts of AGEs.[17] The reaction responsible for the formation of these substances is called the Maillard or browning reaction.[14, 17] Meat is not the only source of AGEs, but meat, cheese, and other high-fat or high-protein foods have the highest amounts of AGEs, while carbs generally have the lowest.[17] Because meats are commonly served in large portions, they are likely to contribute the most overall AGEs. Butter, bacon, oil, beef, and cheese are particularly high in AGEs.[17]

Lean poultry and lean red beef have components in muscle tissue called amino lipids and glucose-6-phosphate, the combination of which rapidly accelerates AGE formation in the presence of heat.[17] Low-fat foods in general, such as whole grains, bread, fruits, low-fat milk, and veggies, are low in AGEs.[17] For example, fried bacon has over ten times the amount of AGEs in two slices when compared with one-third cup of sautéed tofu or baked chicken.[17] Half a cup of roasted chicken has thirty-five times more AGEs than the same amount of red kidney beans.[17]

AGES in Common Foods[17]

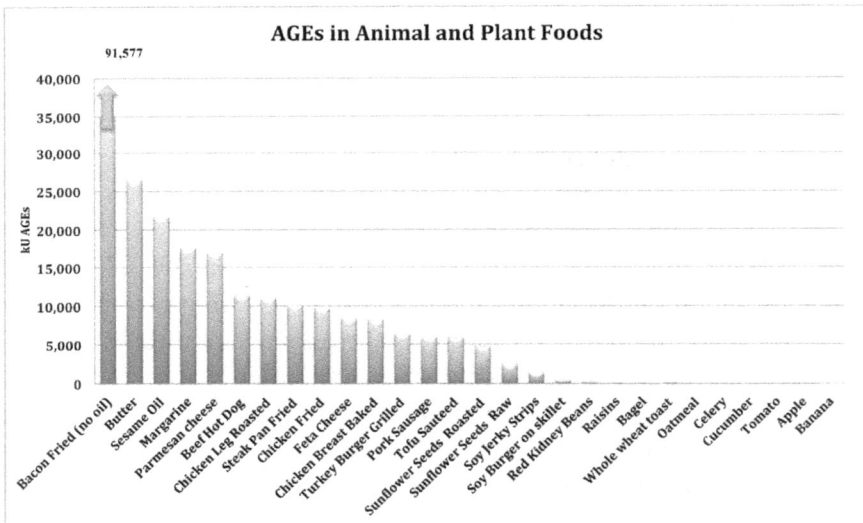

AGEs in Animal and Plant Foods

How to Lower Dietary AGEs

There is no doubt that AGEs are very bad news. Dietary AGEs raise systemic inflammation, which is one major cause of chronic diseases.[17] Dietary intake of AGEs has been implicated in the following diseases:

- Diabetes[14, 17]
- Cardiovascular disease[14, 17]

- Kidney damage [15, 18]
- Pancreatic cancer[19]
- Prostate cancer[20]
- PCOS[21]
- Ovarian dysfunction[22, 23]
- Alzheimer's disease[24–28]
- ALS[25]
- Arthritis[29]
- Asthma[29]
- Cognitive decline[30, 31]
- Crohn's disease[32]
- Barrett's esophagus[33]
- Osteoporosis[34]

What would happen if we lowered the amount of AGEs we eat? It may help prevent diabetes, kidney disease, and heart disease.[29] Reducing AGEs can also accelerate wound healing.[18] Especially for diabetics, decreasing AGEs can make a major difference in inflammatory markers.[31, 35] Low intake of AGEs may even lead to a delay in aging.[18] No wonder some people choose to eat 100% raw foods!

I am not proposing that we all go raw here, but we can definitely try to make some changes to our diets. Adults eat an estimated average of 15,000 units of AGEs per day (kU/day).[18] A diet low in AGEs is therefore one that contains fewer than 15,000 units, and one that is high in AGEs is above 15,000 units. (Keep in mind that just two slices of bacon have 91,577 units of AGEs.[18])

For those of us who are not raw foodists, the first step in lowering dietary AGEs is to cut out fried foods, such as bacon and fried chicken. The second step is to eat more raw fruits and veggies, such as apples, oranges, berries, spinach, and salad greens. This can be done by eating them whole, chopped, juiced, or blended into a smoothie. Finally, eating more whole grains and beans and less meat can help as well. You may be wondering, however, if you will get less protein this way. Again, the reality is that beans have plenty of protein and so do meat substitutes. The concept of a high-protein diet, in general, is questionable for young adults.[11] Seniors above the age of sixty-five may benefit from eating plenty of protein,[11] but why not make it mostly plant protein?

Heme Iron

Iron is an essential nutrient that humans need for good health. Eating enough iron is important for preventing anemia, but eating too much can be a problem. There are two types of iron that we eat: heme iron and nonheme iron.[36] Most of the iron in the food we eat and the supplements we take is nonheme. Meat, fish, shellfish, and seafood contain heme and nonheme iron, while plant foods only have nonheme iron.[36] Clams, mussels, mackerel, pork loin, beef loin, chicken liver, and blood curd (an Asian delicacy) are all rich in heme iron.[36] Red and processed meats such as burgers, sausages, and bacon also contain heme iron. Heme iron is much easier to absorb and store in the body. For the same reason, this kind of iron can be dangerous in excess.[36]

A common blood test used to determine iron stores is called ferritin. Two things that can raise the level of ferritin are iron intake and inflammation. Because there is no way for the body to naturally get rid of the excess, over time, eating too much heme iron raises the ferritin level. Heme iron has a much stronger effect on ferritin levels than nonheme iron.[38-41] Just 5 mg of heme iron per day can make a significant impact on ferritin level.[41] This is important because too much iron can be deadly.[42-47] This accumulation can happen even if you do not have iron overload or hemochromatosis.

Heme Iron Intake and Disease

Year	Author	Subjects	Time	Results
2014	Hunnicutt et al[41]	292,454	10 yr	Heme iron intake was associated with heart disease incidence (nonheme/total iron was inversely associated)
2014	Kaluza et al[42]	36,882	11yr	High heme iron intake increased the risk of fatal heart attacks in men
2013	Kaluza et al[43]	38,859	11 yr	High heme iron intake increased the risk of stroke in men
2013	Fernandez-Cao et al[44]	1073	5 yr	High heme iron intake was associated with an increased risk of developing type 2 diabetes
2012	Genkinger et al[45]	60,895	21 yr	High heme iron and liver intakes increased the risk of endometrial cancer risk by 20-30%
2012	Zhao et al[46]	188,935	Prospective	Heme iron intake was associated with higher risk of type 2 diabetes
1999	Klipstein-Grobusch et al[47]	60	Case/control	Heme iron intake was linked to heart attack in the elderly after adjustment for total calories, fat, saturated fat and cholesterol intake. Strongest link was in former/current smokers, diabetics and adults with high cholesterol who had ferritin> or = 200microg/L.

High-serum ferritin is linked to an increased risk of:

- Diabetes[38–40, 44, 46, 48]
- Insulin resistance[49]
- Hypertension[50]
- Colon cancer[52, 53]
- Multiple myeloma[54]
- Lymphoma[54]
- Acute leukemia[54]
- Lung cancer[55]
- Metabolic syndrome[56]
- Coronary artery disease[57]

Getting more iron than you need is completely unnecessary. The fact is that iron has a proinflammatory effect, which is a bad thing for those trying to prevent the most common chronic diseases. There are many theories as to why or how this excess iron affects the body. Heme iron catalyzes the formation of carcinogenic N-nitroso compounds and toxic aldehydes.[38, 39]

How much is too much iron? Anemia is generally defined as a hemoglobin level below 12 g/dL in women and 13.5 g/dL in men. To make sure these numbers are not too low,[58] doctors often take a look at the hemoglobin and hematocrit tests to check for anemia, but these are not the best indicators of iron storage. Do not count on the regular CBC (complete blood count) test taken at your routine yearly checkup to tell you the whole story.

Asking for a ferritin-level test during a normal checkup can determine if it is too high or too low. A normal ferritin level is generally between 12 ng/mL and 150 ng/mL for women or 300 ng/mL for men,[59] though it would actually be wise to keep ferritin levels below 110 ng/mL for women and below 200 ng/mL for men.[57, 59, 61] Any inflammatory disease can raise ferritin levels,[59] but diabetics, in particular, tend to have an average ferritin level of 44 ng/mL higher than nondiabetics.[61] You can have low iron levels in your blood yet still have very high ferritin because ferritin is elevated with inflammation.

Anemia is not only a result of low iron intake; it may also be due to inflammation that occurs with chronic diseases. This can happen because of diabetes, heart disease, and kidney failure. I have seen lab results from a patient with low iron (34 ug/dL), low hemoglobin (9.6 g/dL), low hematocrit (28.8%), and high ferritin (524 ng/mL). Some kidney failure patients on dialysis even have a ferritin above 800 ng/mL. These numbers reflect the ongoing inflammation that occurs with chronic diseases. However, you can be well within the range of "normal" ferritin levels and still be at a high risk for diabetes or cancer. Check your inflammation level by asking your doctor for an hsCRP test and make sure it is well under 2 mg/L, which can also help decrease the risk of diabetes.[48]

The safest way to eat enough iron without raising ferritin levels too high would be to focus on nonheme sources of iron, such as white beans, spinach, lentils, fortified cereal, and other sources, and limit the heme sources. Avoid beverages like tea or coffee with meals because they can reduce the absorption of iron. Have your doctor check your ferritin levels at least once a year.

Dietary Carcinogens

Grilled, barbecued, and broiled meats have drawbacks not only due to the amount of heme or AGEs in these foods, but also because of carcinogens that form during the cooking process. These are known as heterocyclic amines and polycyclic aromatic hydrocarbons. Heterocyclic amines form when creatine, amino acids, creatinine, and natural sugars in meat react together during cooking.[62-65]

These mutagens in cooked meat are genotoxic, which means that they harm DNA, or genes, in a way that can result in tumor growth.[62] These mutagens are established risk factors of several different types of cancer in humans.[62-68] A combination of these chemicals along with heme iron and AGEs is likely to contribute to the increased risk of cancer associated with excess meat intake.

Different Types of Cancer and Meat Intake

Colon Cancer: Eating pan-fried beefsteak or oven-broiled short ribs or spareribs is associated with an increased risk of colon cancer.[62-64]

Esophageal Cancer: Red meat consumption can double the risk of esophageal cancer.[65]

Gastric (Stomach) Cancer: Consumption of ham, bacon, sausage, and beef contributes to increased gastric cancer risk.[66] An increase of 100 g of red meat intake per day was associated with a 17% increased gastric cancer risk in a recent meta-analysis.[67]

Lung Cancer: Each 120 g of red meat per day can increase the risk of lung cancer by 35%.[68]

Pancreatic Cancer: A high intake of grilled or broiled meat, which contains a concentrated dose of heterocyclic amines, can double the risk of pancreatic cancer in men and raise the risk in women by 29%.[69]

Prostate Cancer: Diets high in saturated fat and well-done meats are linked to advanced prostate cancer.[70]

Rectal Cancer: Poultry cooked at high temperatures may increase the risk of rectal cancer.[64]

Scientists analyzed the US diet and estimated that consumption of meat and fish products may contribute up to 80% of the total cancer risk posed by dietary heterocyclic amines.[71] In a comparison of beef, pork, poultry, game, fish, eggs, and sausage, the highest concentration of heterocyclic amines were detected in pork, game, and chicken breast fried at 200 and 225 degrees.[72] What about heterocyclic amines in plant protein, such as beans and soy products? Though fried tofu and seitan have small amounts of these mutagens, a hamburger cooked under the same conditions has *ten times more* mutagenic activity.[73]

Lowering Cancer Risk with Diet

Diet is very important, but it is not the only factor that causes or affects cancer. Smoking, pollution, alcohol intake, and physical activity can make significant impacts on the incidence of cancer. Regardless of these factors, diet can still make a major impact. What would happen if we reduced or cut out meat and replaced it with more beans and grains as vegetarians often do? Fruits and vegetables are great allies in the fight against cancer, and where we get our protein from is equally important. Of course, not every vegetarian diet is the same, just as all meat eaters do not have the same diet. Still, vegetarians often eat more beans and grains, even if they also eat some junk food. So the mere absence of meat may have some benefits along with an increase in beans and grains.

Can the avoidance of meat lower the risk of cancer or any of the other diseases caused by AGEs, heme iron, and heterocyclic amines?

Some types of cancer are affected more by diet than are others. Most of the current evidence does show that vegetarians have a lower risk of cancer and the other major killer diseases in the United Kingdom and the United States.[74, 75] Vegetarian and vegan diets may lower *stomach* cancer risk by 63%, *multiple myeloma* risk by 77%, and *lymphatic* and *hematopoietic* cancers by 36%.[74] Vegetarians with the highest intakes of veggies, beans, and fiber can nearly cut their risk of *breast* cancer in half.[76] Total cancer incidence in the United Kingdom is 19% lower in vegans, 11% lower in vegetarians, and 12% lower in pescavegetarians/fish eaters.[74] (Some of these numbers may not seem impressive, but again there are other factors involved with cancer, such as smoking, drug consumption, and alcohol intake.) According to a recent study, total cancer incidence in the United States is approximately 16% lower in vegans and 8% lower in vegetarians.[75]

See the *Vegetarian Diet versus Omnivorous Diet* table for evidence that plant-based diets have advantages compared with meat-based diets for cancer prevention and overall mortality.

Vegetarian Diet versus Omnivorous Diet

Year	Location	Authors	Subjects	Findings
2014	UK	Key et al[74]	60,000	Cancer incidence was 19% lower in vegans and 11% lower in vegetarians
2014	UK	Kwok et al[77]	183,000	Heart disease reduced in vegetarian men and women, stroke and mortality reduced in vegetarian men
2014	Spain	Martinez-Gonzalez et al[78]	7,000	Vegetarian diet linked to lower mortality
2014	Austria	Burkert et al[79]	15,000	Vegetarian diet tied to lower vascular risk, lower chronic diseases, higher quality of life compared to carnivorous diet
2013	USA	Orlich et al[80]	73,000	Vegetarian diet reduced all-cause mortality, including reduced heart disease, hypertension, diabetes, and metabolic syndrome
2013	UK	Crowe et al[81]	44,000	Vegetarians had a 32% lower risk of ischemic heart disease
2013	USA	Tantamango et al[73]	69,000	Vegetarian diet protected against cancer
2012	UK/US/Japan	Huang et al[82]	124,000	Vegetarians had a 29% lower heart disease and 18% lower cancer rates
1999	USA	Fraser et al[83]	34,000	Vegetarian men had a 37% reduced risk of heart disease vs non-vegetarians
1998	UK	Key et al[84]	76,000	Vegetarians had a 24% lower risk of death from heart disease

Notes

1. Lin Y, Mouratidou T, Vereecken C, Kersting M, Bolca S, de Moraes AC, et al. "Dietary animal and plant protein intakes and their associations with obesity and cardio-metabolic indicators in European adolescents: the HELENA cross-sectional study." *Nutr* 2015; 14: 10.

2. Lin Y, Bolca S, Vandevijvere S, De Vriese S, Mouratidou T, De Neve M, et al. "Plant and animal protein intake and its association with overweight and obesity among the Belgian population." *Br J Nutr* 2011; 105 (7): 1106-16.

3. Vergnaud AC, Norat T, Romaguera D, Mouw T, May AM, Travier N, et al. "Meat consumption and prospective weight change in participants of the EPIC-PANACEA study." *Am J Clin Nutr* 2010; 92 (2): 398-407.

4. Gilsing AM, Weijenberg MP, Hughes LA, Ambergen T, Dagnelie PC, Goldbohm RA, et al. "Longitudinal changes in BMI in older adults are associated with meat consumption differentially, by type of meat consumed." *J Nutr* 2012; 142 (2): 340-9.

5. Noto H, Goto A, Tsujimoto T, Noda M. "Low carbohydrate diets and all-cause mortaliy: a systematic review and meta-analysis of observational studies." *LoS One* 2013; 8 (1): e55030.

6. Fung TT, van Dam RM, Hankinson SE, Stampfer M, Willett WC, Hu FB. "Low-carbohydrate diets and all-cause and cause-specific mortality: two cohort studies." *Ann Intern Med* 2010; 153 (5): 289-98.

7. Li S, Flint A, Pai JK, Forman JP, Hu FB, Willett WC, Rexrode KM, Mukamal KJ, Rimm EB. "Low carbohydrate diet from plant or animal sources and mortality among myocardial infarction survivors." *J Am Heart Assoc* 2014; 3 (5): e001169.

8. Chen J, Campbell TC Li J, et al. "Diet, lifestyle, and mortality in China. A study of the characteristics of 65 Chinese counties." Oxford, UK; Ithaca, NY; Beijing, PRC: Oxford University Press; Cornell University Press; People's Medical Publishing House, 1990.

9. Guo, WD, Chow WH, Zheng W, Li JY, Blot WJ. "Diet, serum markers and breast cancer mortality in China." *Jpn J Cancer Res* 1994; 85 (6): 572-7.

10. Fontana L, Klein S, Holloszky JO. "Long-term low-protein, low-calorie diet and endurance exercise modulate metabolic factors associated with cancer risk." *Am J Clin Nutr* 2006; 84 (6): 1456-62.

11. Fontana L, Weiss EP, Villareal DT, et al. "Long-term effects of calorie or protein restriction on serum IGF-1 and IGFBP-3 concentration in humans." *Aging Cell* 2008; 7 (5): 681-687.

12. Levine ME, Suarez JA, Brandhorst S, Balasubramanian P, Cheng CW, Madia F, et al. "Low protein intake is associated with a major reduction in IGF-1, cancer, and overall mortality in the 65 and younger but not older population." *Cell Metab* 2014; 19 (3): 407-417.

13. Kim Y, Keogh J, Clifton P. "A review of potential metabolic etiologies of the observed association between red meat consumption and development of type 2 diabetes mellitus." *Metabolism* 2015. [Epub ahead of print]

14. Goldberg T, Cai W, Peppa M, Dardaine V, Baliga BS, Uribarri J, Vlassara H. "Advanced glycoxidation end products in commonly consumed foods." *J Am Diet Assoc* 2004;104(8):1287-91.

15. Uribarri J, Peppa M, Cai W, Goldberg T, Lu M, Baliga S, et al. "Dietary glycotoxins correlate with circulating advanced gylcation end product levels in renal failure patients." *Am J Kidney Dis* 2003; 42 (3): 532-8.

16. Semba RD, Nicklett EJ, Ferrucci L. "Does accumulation of advanced glycation end products contribute to the aging phenotype?" *J Gerontol A Biol Sci Med Sci* 2010; 65A (9): 963-975.

17. Uribarri J, Woodruff S, Goodman S, Cai W, Chen X, Pyzik R, Yong A, Striker GE, Vlassara H. "Advanced glycation end products in foods and a practical guide to their reduction in the diet." *J Am Diet Assoc* 2010; 110 (6): 911-16.

18. Uribarri J, Cai W, Sandu O, Peppa M, Goldberg T, Vlassara H. "Diet-derived advanced glycation end products are major contributors to the body's AGE pool and induce inflammation in healthy subjects." *Ann N Y Acad Sci* 2005; 1043: 461-6.

19. Jiao L, Stolzenberg-Solomon R, Zimmerman TP, Duan Z, Chen L, Kahle L, et al. "Dietary consumption of advanced glycation end

products and pancreatic cancer in prospective NIH-AARP Diet and Health Study." *M J Clin Nutr* 2015; 101 (1): 126-34.

20. Foster D, Spruill L, Walter KR, Noquiera LM, Fedarovich H, Turner RY, et al. "AGE metabolites: a biomarker linked to cancer disparity?" *Cancer Epidemiol Biomarkers Prev* 2014; 23 (10): 2186-91.

21. Merhi Z. "Advanced glycation end products and their relevance in female reproduction." *Hum Reprod* 2014; 29 (1): 135-45.

22. Merhi Z, Mcgee EA, Buyuk E. "Role of advanced glycation end-products in obesity-related ovarian dysfunction." *Minerva Endocrinol* 2014; 39 (3): 167-74.

23. Stensen MH, Tanbo T, Storeng R, Fedorcsak P. "Advanced glycation end products and their receptor contribute to ovarian ageing." *Hum Reprod* 2014; 29 (1): 125-34.

24. Takeuchi M, Kikuchi S, Sasaki N, Suzuki T, Watai T, Iwaki M, Bucala R, Yamagishi S. "Involvement of advanced glycation end-products (AGEs) in Alzheimer's disease." *Curr Alzheimer Res* 2004; 1 (1): 39-46.

25. Sasaki N, Fukatsu R, Tsuzuki K, Hayashi Y, Yoshida T, Fujii N, et al. "Advanced glycation end products in Alzheimer's disease and other neurodegenerative diseases." *Am J Pathol* 1998; 153 (4): 1149-55.

26. Rahmadi A, Steiner N, Munch G. "Advanced glycation endproducts as gerontotoxins and biomarkers for carbonyl-based degenerative processes in Alzheimer's disease." *Clin Chem Lab Med* 2011; 49 (3): 385-91.

27. Srikanth V, Maczurek A, Phan T, Steele M, Wescott B, Juskiw D, et al. "Advanced glycation endproducts and their receptor RAGE in Alzheimer's disease." *Neurobiol Aging* 2011; 32 (5): 763-77.

28. Luevano-Contreras C, Chapman-Novakofski Karen. "Dietary Advanced Glycation End Products and Aging." *Nutrients* 2010; 2 (12): 1247-1265.

29. Chuah YK, Basir R, Talib H, Tie TH, Nordin N. "Receptor for advanced end glycation products and its involvement in inflammatory diseases." *Int J Inflam* (2013), doi:10.1155/2013/403460.

30. Ge X, Xu X, Feng CH, Wang Y, Li YL, Feng B. "Relationships among serum C-reactive protein, receptor for advanced glycation

products, metabolic dyfunction, and cognitive impairments." *BMC Neurol* 2013;13:110.

31. Yaffe K, Lindquist K, Schwartz AV, Vitartas C, Vittinghoff E, Satterfield S, et al. "Advanced glycation end product level, diabetes, and accelerated cognitive aging." *Neurology* 2011; 77 (14): 1351-1356.

32. Ciccocioppo R, Vanoli A, Klersy C, Imbesi V, Boccaccio V, Manca R, et al. "Role of the advanced glycation end products receptor in Crohn's Disease inflammation." *World J Gastroenterol* 2013;19 (45): 8269-8281.

33. Jiao L, Kramer JR, Chen L, Rugge M, Parente P, Verstovsek G, et al. "Dietary consumption of meat, fat, animal products and advanced glycation end-products and the risk of barrett's esophagus." *Aliment Pharmacol Ther* 2013; 38 (7): 10.

34. Yang DH, Chiang TI, Chang IC, Lin FH, Wei CC, Cheng YW. "Increased levels of circulating advanced glycation end-products in menopausal women with osteoporosis." *Int J Med Sci* 2014; 11 (5): 453-60.

35. Vlassara H, Cai W, Crandall J, Goldberg T, Oberstein R, Dardaine V, et al. "Inflammatory mediators are induced by dietary glycotoxins, a major risk factor for diabetic angiopathy." *Proc Natl Acad Sci USA* 2002; 99 (24): 15596-601.

36. Kongkachuichi R, Napatthalung P, Charoensiri R. "Heme and nonheme iron content of animal products commonly consumed in Thailand." 2001; 389-398.

37. Gibson S, Ashwell M. "The association between red and processed meat consumption and iron intakes and status among British adults." *Public Health Nutr* 2003; 6 (4): 341-50.

38. Bao W, Rong Y, Rong S, Liu L. "Dietary iron intake, body iron stores, and risk of type 2 diabetes: a systemic review and meta-analysis." *BMC Med* 2012; 10: 119.

39. Luan de C, Li H, Li SJ, Zhao Z, Li X, Liu ZM. "Body iron stores and dietary iron intake in relation to diabetes in adults in North China." *Diabetes Care* 2008; 31 (2): 285-6.

40. Kunutsor SK, Apekey TA, Walley J, Kain K. "Ferritin levels and risk of type 2 diabetes mellitus: an updated systemic review and

meta-analysis of prospective evidence." *Diabetes Metab Res Rev* 2013; 29 (4): 308-18.

41. Hunnicutt J, He K, Xun P. "Dietary iron intake and body iron stores are associated with risk of coronary heart disease in a meta-analysis of prospective cohort studies." *J Nutr* 2014; 144 (3): 359-66.

42. Kaluza J, Larsson SC, Hakansson N, Wolk A. "Heme iron intake and acute myocardial infarction: a prospective study of men." *J Cardiol* 2014; 172 (1): 155-60.

43. Kaluza J, Wolk A, Larsson SC. "Heme iron intake and risk of stroke: a prospective study of men." *Stroke* 2013; 44 (2): 334-9.

44. Fernandez-Cao JC, Arija V, Bullo M, Basora J, Martinez-Gonzalez MA, Diez-Espino J, Salas-Salvado J. "Heme iron intake and risk of new-onset diabetes in a Mediterranean population at high risk of cardiovascular disease: an observational cohort analysis." *BMC Public Health* 2013; 13: 1042.

45. Genkinger JM, Friberg E, Goldbohm RA, Wolk A. "Long-term dietary heme iron and red meat intake in relation to endometrial cancer risk." *Am J Clin Nutr* 2012; 96 (4): 848-54.

46. Zhao Z, Li S, Liu G, Yan F, Ma X, Huang Z, Tian H. "Body iron stores and heme-iron intake in relation to risk of type 2 diabetes: a systematic review and meta-analysis." *PLoS One* 2012; 7 (7): e41641.

47. Klipstein-Grobusch K, Koster JF, Grobbee DE, Lindemans J, Boeing H, Hofman A, Witteman JC. "Serum ferritin and risk of myocardial infarction in the elderly: the Rotterdam Study." *Am J Clin Nutr* 1999; 69 (6): 1231-6.

48. Andrews Guzman M, Arredondo Olguin M. "Association between ferritin, high sensitivity C-reactive protein (hsCRP) and relative abundance of Hepcidin nRNA with the risk of type 2 diabetes in obese subjects." *Nutr Hosp* 2014; 30 (3): 577-84.

49. Park SK, Choi WJ, Oh CM, Kim MG, Ham WT, Choi JM, Ryoo JH. "Clinical significance of serum ferritin level as an independent predictor of insulin resistance in Korean men." *Diabetes Res Clin Pract* 2015; 107 (1): 187-93.

50. Ryoo JH, Kim SY, Oh CM, Park SK, Kim E, Park SJ, et al. "The incidental relationship between serum ferritin levels and hypertension." *Int Cardiol* 2015; 183: 258-62.
51. Bastide NM, Pierre FH, Corpet DE. "Heme iron from meat and risk of colorectal cancer: a meta-analysis and a review of the mechanisms involved." *Cancer Prev Res* (Phila) 2011; 4 (2): 177-84.
52. Kim E, Coelho D, Blachier F. "Review of the association between meat consumption and risk of colorectal cancer." *Nutr Res* 2013; 33 (12): 983-94.
53. Balder HF, Vogel J, Jansen MC, Weijenberg MP, van den Brandt PA, Westerbrink S, et al. "Heme and chlorophyll intake and risk of colorectal cancer in the Netherlands cohort study." *Cancer Epidemiol Biomarkers Prev* 2006; 15 (4): 717-25.
54. Zhang XZ, Su AL, Hu MQ, Zhang XQ, Xu YL. "Elevated serum ferritin levels in patients with hematologic malignancies." *Asian Pac J Cancer Prev* 2014; 15 (15): 6099-101.
55. Ji M, Li XD, Shi HB, Ning ZH, Zhao WQ, Wang Q, et al. "Clinical significance of serum ferritin in elderly patients with primary lung carcinoma." *Tumour Biol* 2014; 35 (10): 10195-9.
56. Abril-Ulloa V, Flores-Mateo G, Sola-Alberich R, Manuel-y-Keenoy B, Arija V. "Ferritin levels and risk of metabolic syndrome: a meta-analysis of observational studies." *MC Public Health* 2014; 14: 483.
57. Pourmoghaddas A, Sanei H, Garakyaraghi M, Esteki-Ghashghaei F, Gharaati M. "The relation between body iron store and ferritin, and coronary artery disease." *ARYA Atheroscler* 2014; 10 (1): 32-6.
58. "Anemia", American Society of Hematology, Accessed May 1, 2015, http://www.hematology.org/Patients/Anemia/.
59. "Ferritin Blood Test", MedlinePlus, U.S. National Library of Medicine, Accessed May 1, 2015, http://www.nlm.nih.gov/medlineplus/ency/article/003490.htm.
60. Montonen J, Boeing H, Steffen A, Lehmann R, Fritsche A, Joost HG, et al. "Body iron stores and risk of type 2 diabetes: a result from the European Prospective Investigation into Cancer and Nutrition (EPIC)-Potsdam study." *Diabetologia* 2012; 55 (10): 2613-21.

61. Orban E, Schwab S, Thorand B, Huth C. "Association of iron indices and type 2 diabetes: a meta-analysis of observational studies." *Diabetes Metab Res Rev* 2014; 30 (5): 372-94.

62. Joshi AD, Kim A, Lewinger JP, Ulrich CM, Potter JD, Cotterchio M, et al. "Meat intake, cooking methods, dietary carcinogens, and colorectal cancer risk: findings from the Colorectal Cancer Family Registry." *Cancer Med* 2015. [Epub ahead of print]

63. Wang J, Joshi AD, Corral R, Siegmund KD, Marchand LL, Martinez ME, et al. "Carcinogenic metabolism genes, red meat and poultry intake, and colorectal cancer risk." *Int J Cancer* 2012; 130 (8): 1898-907.

64. Ollberding NJ, Wilkens LR, Henderson BE, Kolonel LN, Marchland LL. "Meat consumption, heterocyclic amines, and colorectal cancer risk: The Multiethnic Cohort Study." *Int J Cancer* 2012; 131 (7): E1125-E1133.

65. Golozar A, Eternadi A, Kamanger F, Fazeltabar Malekshah A, Islami F, Nasrollahzadeh D, et al. "Food preparation methods, drinking water source, and esophageal squamous cell carcinoma in the high-risk area of Golestan, Northeast Iran." *Eur J Cancer Prev* 2015. [Epub ahead of print]

66. Zhu H, Yang X, Zhang C, Zhu C, Tao G, Zhao L, et al. "Red and processed meat intake is associated with higher gastric cancer risk: a meta-analysis of epidemiological observational studies." *PLoS One* 2013; 8 (8): e70955.

67. Song P, Lu M, Yin Q, Zhang D, Fu B, Wang B, Zhao Q. "Red meat consumption and stomach cancer risk: a meta-analysis." *J Cancer Res Clin Oncol* 2014; 140 (6): 979-92.

68. Xue XJ, Gao Q, Qiao JH, Zhang J, Xu CP, Liu J. "Red and processed meat consumption and the risk of lung cancer: a dose response meta-analysis of 33 published studies." *Int J Clin Exp Med* 2014; 7 (6): 1542-53.

69. Stolzenberg-Solomon RZ, Cross AJ, Silverman DT, Schairer C, Thompson FE, Kipnis V, et al. "Meat and meat-mutagen intake and pancreatic cancer risk in the NIH-AARP cohort." *Cancer Epidemiol Biomarkers Prev* 2007; 16 (12): 2664-75.

70. Gathirua-Mwangi WG, Zhang J. "Dietary factors and risk for advanced prostate cancer." *Eur J Cancer Prev* 2014; 23 (2): 96-109.

71. Layton DW, Bogen KT, Knize MG, Hatch FT, Johnson VM, Felton JS. "Cancer risk of heterocyclic amines in cooked foods: an analysis and implications for research." *Carcinogenesis* 1995; 16 (1): 39-52.

72. Skog K, Augustsson K, Steineck G, Stenberg M, Jagerstad M. "Polar and non-polar heterocyclic amines in cooked fish and meat products and their corresponding pan residues." *Food Chem Toxicol* 1997; 35 (6): 555-65.

73. Knize MG, Dolbeare FA, Cunninham PL, Felton JS. "Mutagenic activity and heterocyclic amine content of the human diet." *Princess Takamatsu Symp* 1995; 23: 30-8.

74. Key TJ, Appleby PN, Crowe FL, Bradbury KE, Schmidt JA, Travis RC. "Cancer in British vegetarians: updated analyses of 4998 incident cancers in a cohort of 32,491 meat eaters, 8612 fish eaters, 18,298 vegetarians, and 2246 vegans." *Am J Clin Nutr* 2014; 100 Suppl 1: 378s-85s.

75. Tantamango-Bartley Y, Jaceldo-Siegl K, Fan J, Fraser G. "Vegetarian diets and the incidence of cancer in a low-risk population." *Cancer Epidemiol Biomarkers Prev* 2013; 22: 286-94.

76. Dos Santos Silva I, Mangtani P, McCormack V, Bhakta D, Sevak L, McMichael AJ. "Lifelong vegetarianism and risk of breast cancer: a population-based case-control study among South Asian migrant women living in England." *Int J Cancer* 2002; 99 (2): 238-44.

77. Kwok CS, Umar S, Myint PK, Mamas MA, Loke YK. "Vegetarian diet, Seventh Day Adventists and risk of cardiovascular mortality: a systematic review and meta-analysis." *Int J Cardiol* 2014; 176 (3): 680-6.

78. Martinez-Gonzalez MA, Sanchez-Tainta A, Corella D, Salas-Salvado J, Ros E, Aros F, et al. "A provegetarian food pattern and reduction in total mortality in the Prevencion con Dieta Mediterranea (PREDIMED) study." *Am J Clin Nutr* 2014; 100 Suppl 1: 320s-8s.

79. Burkert NT, Freidl W, Grossschadel F, Muckenhuber J, Stronegger WJ, Rasky E. "Nutrition and health: different forms of diet and

their relationship with various health parameters among Austrian adults." *Wien Klin Wochenschr* 2014; 126 (3-4): 113-8.

80. Orlich MJ, Fraser GE. "Vegetarian diets in the Adventist Health Study 2: a review of initial published findings." *Am J Clin Nutr* 2014; 100 Suppl 1: 353s-8s.

81. Crowe FL, Appleby PN, Travis RC, Key TJ. "Risk of hospitalization or death from ischemic heart disease among British vegetarians and nonvegetarians: results from the EPIC-Oxford cohort study." *Am J Clin Nutr* 2013; 97 (3): 597-603.

82. Huang T, Yang B, Zheng J, Li G, Wahlqvist ML, Li D. "Cardiovascular disease mortality and cancer incidence in vegetarians: a meta-analysis and systemic review." *Ann Nutr Metab.* 2012; 60 (4): 233-40.

83. Fraser GE. "Diet as primordial prevention in Seventh-Day Adventists." *Prev Med* 1999; 29 (6 Pt 2): s18-23.

84. Key TJ, Fraser GE, Thorgood M, Appleby PN, Beral V, Reeves G, etal. "Mortality in vegetarians and non-vegetarians: a collaborative analysis of 8300 deaths among 76,000 men and women in five prospective studies." *Public Health Nutr* 1998; 1 (1): 33-41.

CHAPTER 10

My Life and Health

Nearly two decades ago, my favorite foods were pepperoni pizza, hot dogs, filet mignon, and fried mozzarella sticks. Much like the average American, I often enjoyed a good bacon and egg breakfast. I recall my mother teaching me to make scrambled eggs mixed with cheese. This was one of the first meals that I learned to cook. So what happened to change my mind about all these foods? How is it possible that I can now live without eating any of them?

Everything changed after I stayed on a farm in Germany for an exchange program arranged by my middle school. It was a farm in a remote village with cows, pigs, chickens, and rabbits. One day, I asked my exchange student why she kept the rabbits in the back of the yard and if they were her pets. She said that the rabbits were not pets at all. Her grandmother would eventually eat them. This was so shocking to me because I had pet rabbits back home in Florida. At the time, I could not imagine eating a pet rabbit just as I could not imagine eating my dog today.

The problem is that her logic was not flawed. I came to realize that my logic was the one with obvious flaws. I thought about how we choose to eat certain animals and yet others are treated as family members. Most people do not realize that farm animals can be intelligent and sentient individuals.

I wanted to change my diet and set out to do just that when I returned home. My parents, however, were very worried about this sudden change of heart. They, not unlike the majority of Americans at the time, believed that children need meat to survive, grow, and develop into healthy adults. My dad is a bacon-loving, steak-and-potatoes kind of man. He knew that I enjoyed those foods as well so it was a surprise when I no longer wanted them. Since I was only thirteen years old, cutting out meat from my diet seemed an extreme transition. They told me that I might get sick and possibly even stop growing.

My father wanted to make sure that my decision was based on quality information and facts. He said, "If you are going to do this, then you will do it right." He bought a stack of books about the vegetarian diet and nutrition in general. My parents probably thought it was a phase and that it might discourage me. I was learning about nutrition and how it affected diseases virtually burying myself in the books. At the time, I did not feel discouraged, it actually fascinated me. I read all of these books and bought several more. I found that many of my beliefs about food, much like those of my friends and family members, were based on numerous myths and not scientific evidence. Initially, I became a vegetarian because of ethics but this quickly changed into a decision based on scientific evidence and logic.

My mother started calling local doctors and nutritionists to evaluate my health and my diet. She thought that I would suffer from a nutrient deficiency so she had them take my blood, run several tests, and evaluate it. After my blood was tested and analyzed, a doctor at the lab called my mother and said that I would live to be 170 years old according to the test results! Not only was I free of any kind of deficiency but also my lipids and cholesterol levels were very low just as they remain today—almost two decades later.

The truth, of course, is that we do not need to eat meat to survive. Not only does modern research support the benefits of a diet low in meat but it also shows that completely eliminating meat from one's diet can be beneficial, as discussed in the previous chapters. I have personally reaped a long list of benefits from eating a strictly plant-based diet. This lifestyle has kept my weight, body fat, blood pressure, cholesterol, and triglycerides low. I have never suffered from iron deficiency or any other major health problem before.

What about strength and muscles? How can I possibly maintain or grow muscle just by eating plants? This question was already partially addressed in the protein chapter (chapter 7). Despite plenty of research to the contrary, there is a stereotype that vegans are weak and cannot build muscle as readily as meat eaters can. The fact is that building muscle on a diet made of plants is not difficult. I have plenty of muscle and I do not take supplements, or use powders or protein shakes. My protein intake is made mostly of beans, whole grains, tofu, tempeh, nuts, seeds and some soy-based meat alternatives. When I have plenty of time, I germinate and cook beans combined with veggies in a stew or soup. I try to focus on whole foods as often as possible. When I am in a hurry, though, I might warm up a veggie burger or soy-based "chicken" strips to top a salad, for example.

Photo from 1996

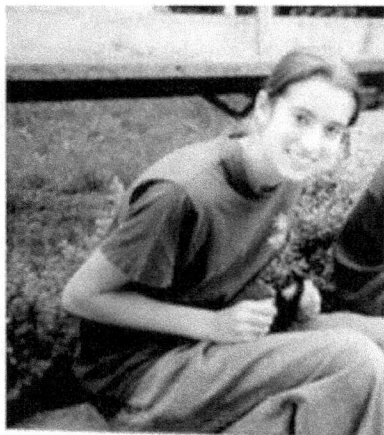

Photo from 2015

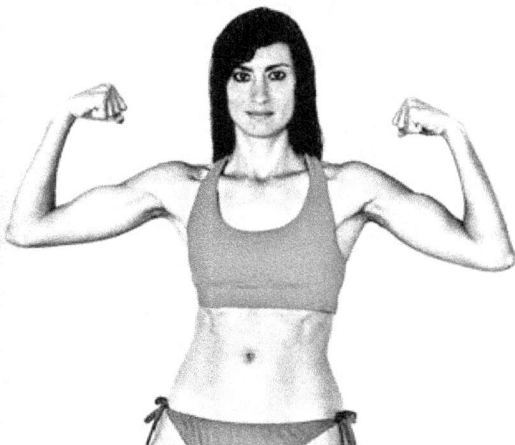

This is a photo of me holding a baby bunny in Germany. I was 12 years old.

This is a photo of me at 31 years old.

My fitness level is similar to or even better than that of many of my peers when it comes to strength or cardio-type workouts. Most women cannot do a regular pull-up, and I am proud to say that I can. I can also bicep curl a 20-lb weight on each arm, while my female friends can barely handle 15-lb dumbbells. I have joined intense hour-long cycling classes at the gym and made it through the whole workout even after I have gone months without really exercising. I survived a very intense strength work-out resulting in nothing more than severe muscle soreness for a few days while a younger friend of mine was hospitalized with a very swollen arm after doing the same type of routine. Coincidentally, this friend was eating a low carb caveman-style diet at the time.

As far as body mass index (BMI) and body fat go, I have always been on the low side, but my diet has definitely helped maintain that as I have seen so many friends and family members continue to gain weight as they age. BMI is a rough estimate of body fat using a ratio of weight to height ([wt in kg]^2/[ht in meters]^2). My body fat is 20% while the average fe-male American has 40% body fat.[1] This is due to the fact that most are overweight or obese. What about normal-weight women? Normal-weight women have a body fat of 34% on average.[1] If eating meat is so important for growing and maintaining muscle, then I would have less muscle and more fat than the average meat-eating woman. The reality is that more of my weight is muscle and less is fat, even when compared to many women with normal body weights.

What does it mean to have 34% or 40% body fat? According to these numbers, a woman that weighs 140 lb (my weight) would have 56 lb of fat (40% fat) instead of my 28 lb of fat, because I have 20% body fat. The aver-age woman, in other words, has double the body fat that I have. For those of normal weight with 34% body fat, each would have 47 lb of fat, which is still nearly 20 lb more fat when compared to my body composition.

My Conclusion

Why did I share all these details about my life? Simply to share some of the benefits and struggles that can accompany plant-based eating. I still feel that food ethics are important, however, following nutrition facts remains the force that drives my passion. Eating a diet that is very different from what friends and family eat can be taxing because of all the comments or criticisms. My family was very worried that my health would suffer when I first eliminated meat from my diet. Now, eighteen years later, they are convinced that I made a healthy choice and even venture to taste some of my meals. Many friends have completely changed and remain vegan today. This includes two former boyfriends, one of whom has been vegan for over twelve years. My husband was the kind of person who makes fun of vegans but now he is one. Despite being in the military surrounded by a machismo driven culture, he has remained a vegan for several years. He feels that it is not the most difficult change he has ever made. Overall, about 5% of Americans consider themselves vegetarian, which is over 16 million people.[2, 3]

Most people who go vegetarian or vegan lose weight. Unfortunately, not everyone will experience the exact same effects even if they eat the same foods. Genes still play a role in health, but bad genes do not necessarily mean a death sentence. Diet and lifestyle make a big difference, no matter what kind of genes you have. Looking at my health alongside all of the research in previous chapters, it is clear that people who eat the plant-based way tend to experience similar health benefits, regardless of genetic background. While I cannot guarantee that eating this way will solve all of your health problems, I can say that you will never know until you try it!

If you are adamantly opposed to giving up bacon and steak then simply set a goal to try new plant foods each week. You do not have to make a radical change "cold turkey" if the thought is too overwhelming. I was the kind of person who loved bacon and steak many years ago, and now I would not dream of eating either. I was able to cut all of it out and still enjoy my meals. Fruits and veggies were not my favorites as a young child, but I love them now more than ever! Keep in mind that taste buds change over time. Give yours time to adapt.

Notes:

1. M. P. St-Onge, "Are normal-weight Americans over-fat?" *Obesity (Silver Spring)*, 18 (2010): 2067–8.

2. "In U.S. 5% Consider Themselves Vegetarians," Frank Newport, Gallup Poll, Accessed August 19, 2015, http://www.gallup.com/poll/156215/consider-themselves-vegetarians.aspx.

3. United States Census Bureau, Accessed August 19, 2015, http://www.census.gov/

CHAPTER 11

The Anti-Caveman Diet

Current research—much of it described in this book—suggests that the modern version of the caveman diet is not only unhealthy but may also actually increase the risk of multiple chronic diseases, especially in those who eat plenty of red meat. The opposite of low carb, or Anti-Caveman, would be to eat more beans and grains while reducing or eliminating meat. This Anti-Caveman diet goes against the low-carb principles set by Paleo pundits because it turns out to be a high-carb diet (not to be confused with a high-calorie diet). Most sources of plant protein also contain plenty of complex carbs.

Everyone can agree that it's important to eat more fruits and veggies, but after seeing all of the issues with meat, one must question whether we should be eating meat at every meal or even every day. Since humans can get all the protein they need from beans and whole grains, it is difficult to nutritionally justify the need to eat meat every day. You may benefit from reducing meat intake to less than once a day. Perhaps it is time to ask yourself some hard questions. How often do you crave meat? Do you feel a desire to eat it at every meal? Every day? Every week? Or can you simply save meat for special occasions like dinner at a friend's house, parties, or family gatherings?

Based on all the evidence presented in this book, humans can benefit from reducing meat intake and replacing much of it with alternative protein sources. Bacon, ham, burgers, and hot dogs should probably be reserved for special occasions or avoided entirely. Beans, nuts, and whole grains, on the other hand, should be a part of most meals. Fake meat and real processed meats are both processed foods. But processed soy burgers and soy hot dogs are better alternatives to real hot dogs and real hamburgers because soy meats are lower in saturated fat, cholesterol, AGEs, heme iron, heterocyclic amines, and other harmful substances. Another advantage is that soy burgers tend to have some fiber while real burgers and hot dogs have none.

Some people are perfectly happy without any meat, and some only desire it once a week. You can decide which option is easiest to fit your lifestyle, but whatever you decide, at least you now have more nutritional knowledge to empower you to make healthy choices.

The Anti-Caveman Diet
What is the Anti-Caveman Diet?

- Aim for 90–100% plant-based foods
- At least 80% whole foods/low in processed foods
- Rich in omega-3
- High in fiber and natural carbs
- Low in saturated fat
- Low in cholesterol

The Anti-Caveman diet is comprised of mostly whole-plant foods. It is a high-fiber, plant-based diet with an emphasis on whole grains, nuts, and legumes for protein in addition to generous daily doses of veggies, fruits, seeds, and seaweed. This diet is not necessarily 100% whole foods because it does include small amounts of oil and whole-grain cereal/bread/pasta, soy yogurt, almond milk, and other relatively healthy processed foods, which make meals fast and convenient when time is limited. See *Daily*

Average Anti-Caveman Diet Recommendations for general Anti-Caveman diet recommendations and suggestions. Meeting these recommendations results in a total of about 1350 calories and 55 grams of protein leaving room for larger serving sizes and some additional foods for individuals who need more calories.

Daily Average Anti-Caveman Diet Recommendations (Amounts will vary from person to person. Use less oil if possible.)

Basic Food Guide

Food	Priority	Total	Examples
Vegetables	Essential	3 cups	Spinach, Kale, Collards
Fruits	Essential	2 cups	Grapes, Berries, Pears
Beans	Essential	1.5 cups	Black, Kidney, Lentils
Whole Grains	Essential	1.5 cups	Oats, Brown Rice, Quinoa
Nuts/Seeds	Essential	1 oz	Walnuts, Chia, Flax
Sea Vegetables	Essential	1 Tbsp	Nori, Dulse, Wakame
Non-Dairy	Optional	2 cups	Almond milk, Soymilk
Oil	Optional	2 Tbsp	Flax oil, Canola oil
Meat Alternative	Optional	½ cup	Tofu, Veggie burger
Condiments	Optional	2 Tbsp	Agave, Nutritional yeast
Supplements	According to Blood Test Results	1 dose each (per test results)	Vit D, Vit B12, DHA

The Anti-Caveman diet includes some processed foods such as tofu, whole-wheat bread, whole-grain pasta, flax oil, agave, and nondairy cheese. Making meals convenient is one of the top priorities for families and single people alike. The fact is that convenience drives people to buy fast food among other types of junk foods. An exclusively whole-food diet without oil or anything processed is healthy but may be very difficult and time-consuming in practice. The same goes for a totally raw diet, in which homemade meals only last for a day or two before spoilage and changes in flavor occur. Unfortunately, fresh and raw foods are quick to spoil, so using some processed and fortified foods can make proper nutrition much more convenient.

The main goal is not only to eat more vegetables, fruit, whole grains, and beans but also to enjoy eating these foods. Some people need comfort foods at least once a week. This is why I do not suggest completely removing all added oil or sweeteners from the diet. Making veggies taste good is fast and easy when you can add small amounts of oil, sauce, or other minimally processed foods. The same concept goes for making green shakes or desserts with small amounts of natural sweeteners, such as agave or maple syrup.

Some nutrients of concern for those used to eating an average American diet are magnesium, potassium, fiber, vitamin D, and omega-3 fat. Vitamin D and omega-3 fat also tend to be low in the average vegetarian and vegan diets. For vegetarians/vegans, the nutrients to be mindful of, in addition to vitamin D and omega-3 fat, are vitamin B_{12}, iron, zinc, and calcium. These nutrients are not hard to find in plant foods, but they are often overlooked with a diet of mostly processed foods. A plant-based diet can provide sufficient amounts of these and other nutrients with the following foods:

Anti-Caveman Essential Examples

- Calcium: spinach, chard, kale
- Iodine: seaweed (e.g., nori, dulse, wakame)
- Iron: beans, greens; use cast-iron cookware daily
- Omega-3 (ALA): chia seeds, flaxseeds, walnuts
- Omega-3 (EPA/DHA): DHA microalgae vegan supplements (an environmentally friendly alternative to fish oil). The body can efficiently convert ALA to EPA but not to DHA.
- Selenium: brazil nuts
- Vitamin D: sunshine (expose 75% of skin daily for short periods of time) or vitamin D supplements
- Vitamin B_{12}: fortified soy milk, fortified almond milk, fortified cereal, vitamin supplements
- Probiotics: miso, kimchi, soy yogurt, kombucha
- Zinc: pumpkin seeds, cashews

Improving health is all about looking at the big picture, not about nit-picking at protein, gluten, carbs, fat, or oil. Of course, refined and processed carbs like soda and candy are not helpful for weight loss or overall health. We can all do with adding more fruits and veggies to our diets while reducing junk food like candy, chips, and soda. But cutting out high-fiber carbs, like beans and whole grains, while increasing meat intake does more damage than good for all of the reasons described in the past few chapters. This is why eating more complex carbs can actually help improve health. So the goal should be to use beans, nuts, seeds, and grains as the main protein source, and if desired, occasionally indulge in meat or other animal products. This is both a great strategy for weight loss and an anti-inflammatory diet. Using this goal can make a high daily fiber intake of 40–50 g realistic and achievable, though this is much higher than the usual US intake of 16 g. Another important aspect is a low ratio of omega-6 to omega-3 fat, which can be achieved with the inclusion of flaxseeds, chia seeds, walnuts, and algal DHA.

The Best Kind of Fat

Americans eat too much omega-6 and not enough omega-3 fat, which can lead to inflammation. How do you get essential fat on a plant-based diet if you don't eat fish? Many plant fats and oils have essential fatty acids, including omega-6 and omega-3. Omega-3 is anti-inflammatory, but it is only found in a limited number of foods. Most oils have a small amount of omega-3 fat.

Vegetable oil, which is usually just soybean oil (read the label on the oil you cook with), is mostly omega-6 fat, so it is not a good source of omega-3. Olive oil is not a good source of omega-3 or omega-6 because it is mostly *monounsaturated* fat, which is heart healthy but not an essential fat. Flaxseed oil and fish oil are rich in omega-3 fat. Both of those options are very expensive with distinctly fishy flavors. These two oils may be healthy, but they are not practical for cooking purposes.

Both olive oil and canola oil are relatively inexpensive cooking oils compared with, for example, coconut oil. Coconut oil is a saturated fat. It is not a good source of *essential* fatty acids, despite its recent popularity. Olive oil and canola oil are high in monounsaturated fat. Olive oil contains only

1% omega-3 fat. Canola oil has nine times more omega-3 fat than olive oil, and the ratio of omega-6 to omega-3 fat in canola oil is 2 to 1 versus 10 to 1 in olive oil. (See focus on Omega-3 Fat charts)

Focus on Omega-3 Fat

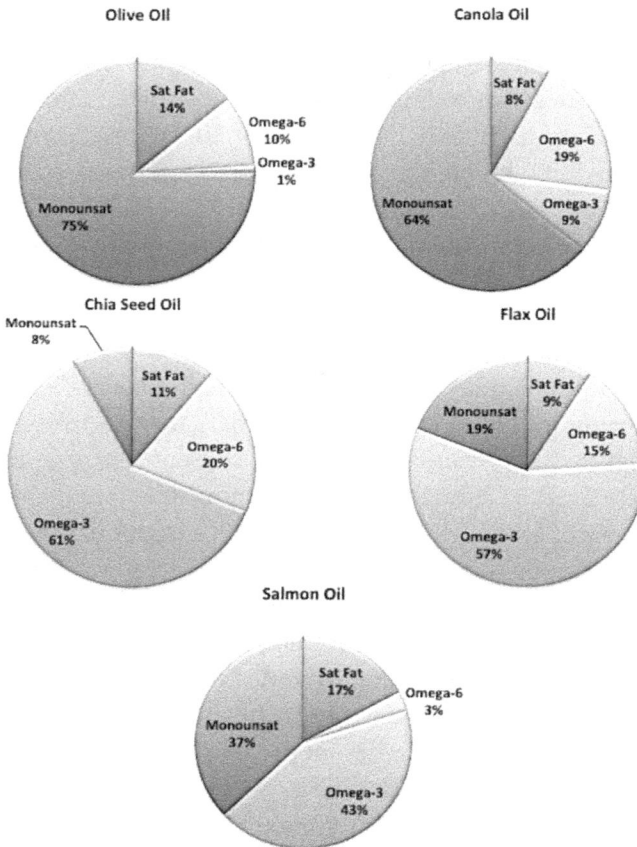

Data compiled by Jen Swallow from US Department of Agriculture, Agricultural Research Service. 2014. USDA National Nutrient Database for Standard Reference, Release 27. Nutrient Data Laboratory home page, http://www.ars.usda.gov/nutrientdata.

Substituting canola for olive oil works fine in most recipes and can help increase the total amount of omega-3 in any diet. The best plant-based sources of omega-3 are flaxseed and chia seeds, which are, proportionally, even higher than fish in omega-3 fat. More than half of the total fat in both flaxseed and chia seeds is omega-3 fat, compared with 43% in salmon. Salmon has more saturated and monounsaturated fat when compared with flax and chia. Salmon also has a mixture of long chain and medium chain omega-3 fat, while seeds do not have long chain omega-3 fat. This is why it is important to take an algal oil (vegan) omega-3 supplement for those who do not eat fish. Algae oil has long chain omega-3 fat.

Why Not Try 100% Plant Based?

Taking the focus away from a meat-centered diet, such as Paleo, and moving toward a balanced plant-based diet, such as a vegetarian or vegan diet, can be a big transition for many people, but it is worth all the effort. (See chapter 4 for a list of large research studies showing that vegans and vegetarians are consistently slimmer than meat eaters.) For this and many more reasons, a growing population has chosen to replace meat with plant protein. Vegetarians and vegans have long reaped the numerous health benefits of this choice.[1-6] This does not mean that being mostly vegetarian with an occasional indulgence in meat would not have any benefits. Doing your best to get close to 90–100% plant based, however, can pay off in the long run. A healthy vegetarian diet can lower weight, blood pressure, cholesterol, total to HDL cholesterol ratio, triglycerides, and the probability of coronary heart disease.[1]

What can you expect to see if you go 100% strictly plant-based?

- Permanent weight loss/low BMI[1, 2]
- Lower blood pressure[3]
- Lower total cholesterol[2-4]
- Lower LDL cholesterol[2, 4-7]

- Lower triglycerides[2, 4]
- Lower inflammation[8]

What This Diet Has Done for Me

Not all vegetarian or vegan diets are healthy or even alike. There are whole-food, raw-food, oil-free, and junk-food vegans with very different diets. People can call themselves vegans while living on french fries, soda, and candy. Some vegans admit that they do not eat vegetables. This is not the way to achieve any of the health benefits described in this book. The Anti-Caveman diet, which is modeled after my personal diet, is a specific plant-based diet with plenty of vegetables, fruits, beans, whole grains, nuts, and seeds, plus a small proportion of processed foods for convenience and taste. The point of this diet is not to give up everything you enjoy, but rather to focus on healthy foods and still enjoy every meal. The Anti-Caveman diet is, therefore, not oil-free or 100% whole foods, but it aims to reduce processed foods and added oils.

There are significant differences between vegetarians and vegans in terms of health benefits.[9–15] These differences are often reflected in weight status and blood test results. Some people are vegetarian or vegan, yet still eat plenty of junk food with few vegetables or fruits. Emphasizing whole foods instead of processed foods is the most important factor in determining success with any diet, not just vegan or vegetarian diets. I have firsthand experience as to how a strict plant-based diet can keep all of these risk factors low and maintain good health. See how my health, after being on the Anti-Caveman diet for eighteen years, compares with that of others in the *Sample Labs Recorded in Past Studies versus My Labs* table.[16] (Again, not all vegan diets are the same; some enjoy better health than others.)

Sample Labs Recorded in Past
Studies versus My Labs

Tests	Meat eater	Vegetarian	Vegan	My Results 2014
Blood Pressure	127/78[9]	123/73[9]	123/71[9]	105/66
Total Cholesterol	200[10]	188[4] (in UK)	172[4] (in UK)	111
LDL Cholesterol (Bad)	120[11]	99[13]	88[14]	50
HDL Cholesterol (Good)	50[11]	43[13]	51[15]	51
Triglycerides	120[11]	46[13]	71[15]	50
CRP (Inflammation)	1.6[12]	N/A	N/A	<0.5

Eliminating all or most animal products from one's diet is extreme enough for most people, so there is no need to further restrict the diet by cutting oil or faux meats (unless you are instructed by a clinician to do so). Simply adding a daily regimen of fruits, veggies, beans, and whole grains can make a big difference in health. The Anti-Caveman diet is more about reducing animal products and relying mostly on plant protein and less about giving up the foods you love. The closer you can get to 100% plant foods, the better.

What about fish? Or chicken? How does a pescatarian diet (includes fish) or semivegetarian diet (includes chicken and fish) compare with the vegan diet since they often include small or moderate amounts of meat? Low-meat diets like these do confer several health benefits, but they do not have quite the same protection against weight gain or obesity. See the table below for a comparison of weight status/BMI between different types of diets.

Different Types of Diets and Weight Status

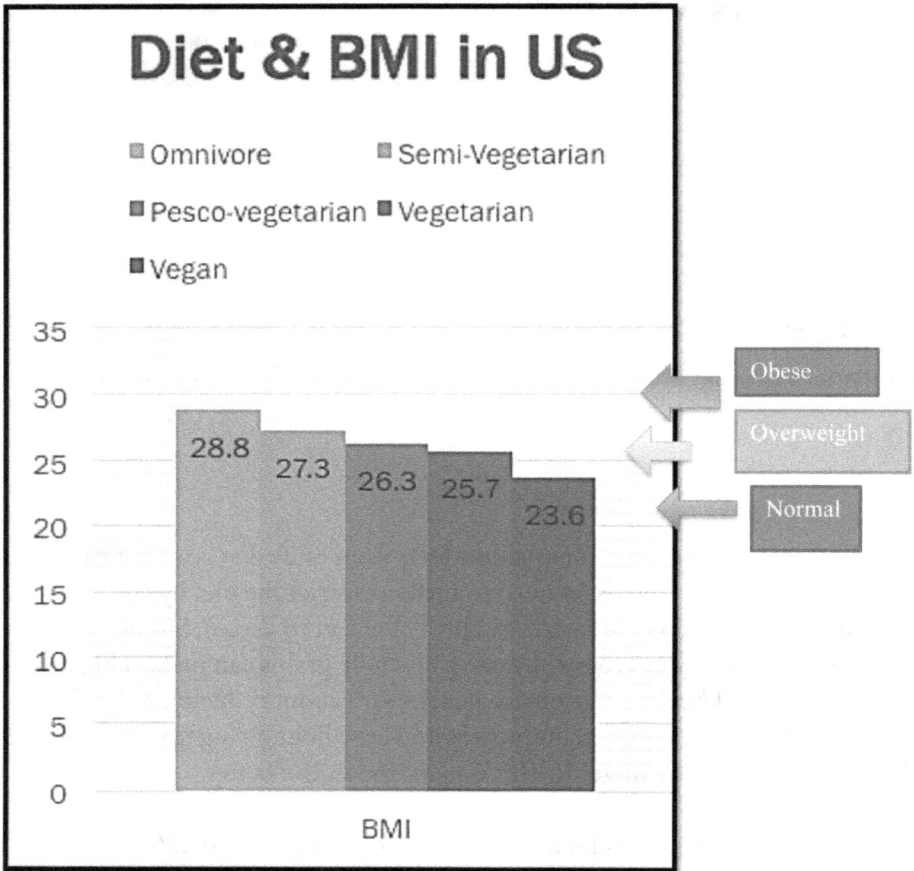

Diet & BMI in US

◾ Omnivore ◾ Semi-Vegetarian

◾ Pesco-vegetarian ◾ Vegetarian

◾ Vegan

Obese

Overweight

Normal

28.8
27.3
26.3
25.7
23.6

BMI

The average weight status of vegans shows that a high fiber diet that is very low in saturated fat tends to keep people thin. In the long-term, vegan and vegetarian diets are effective for reaching and maintaining a healthy weight.[17] Compared with vegans, omnivores have double the prevalence of being overweight, which is a BMI above 24.9, and quadruple the prevalence of obesity, which is a BMI above 30.[17] On average, American vegans are at a normal weight (BMI 23.6), while meat eaters are overweight (BMI 28.7).[17]

Evaluate Your Health Objectively over Time

When it comes to your health, it's crucial to monitor changes as early as possible. Put yourself in the driver's seat; don't simply act as a passenger watching and waiting for accidents to happen. Just because you think you feel healthy does not mean you are healthy. Once a year, have your blood tested at your doctor's office and keep a file with the results so that you can track changes over time. It is never too early to start. I have seen patients in their teens with high cholesterol. Ask for a printout of these labs every year:

- Hemoglobin
- Hematocrit
- Ferritin
- Total cholesterol
- LDL cholesterol
- HDL cholesterol
- Triglycerides
- Homocysteine
- Hs CRP
- ESR
- HbA1c
- Vitamin D
- Vitamin B$_{12}$

Caveman Conclusion

Remember that you're not a caveman. Cavemen did not have all of the choices that we have today. They lived in a world so unlike ours. It was a world completely lacking the indulgence we see today. Maintaining a healthy weight is a struggle in this fast-paced culture of convenience. We are surrounded by junk food at every turn. The first and last items we see upon entering or exiting a grocery store are chips, pastries, and candy. Fast food burgers and fried chicken are available at nearly every exit off of major highways. Most Americans continue to indulge in these foods and even feed them to children.

The norm in this country is to eat fast food, chips, and processed meat and drink soda on a daily basis. Even in a place that promotes health and wellness, such as a hospital, finding a fast-food restaurant in the lobby is not uncommon. If there is no McDonald's or Wendy's in the building, employees still find a way to bring burgers, soda, and fries to work.

Despite all of these unhealthy habits, Americans often feel as if they are helpless victims of preventable diseases like hypertension, obesity, or heart disease. People turn to magazine articles, family anecdotes, TV shows, and blogs rather than reading a nutrition textbook or speaking with a licensed nutrition professional. There are so many steps we can take toward a better lifestyle. Can you imagine if every office had a bowl of fresh fruit instead of candy sitting on each desk? This seems like a strange idea, but it is a logical step in the right direction.

Carbs are constantly demonized in the media because we all know that cookies and cake are unhealthy. Yet most people still believe that meat should be the center of every meal. The vast amount of data included in this book has shown that eating meat two or three times a day is not a healthy way to go. In reality, meat should be treated more like other rich and unhealthy foods because we do not need to eat it every day. If you do not eat French fries, cookies or cake with every meal then you should not eat meat with every meal. Meat should be considered a treat.

When it comes to your health, ignorance is not bliss. Take control of your health and stop depending on other people to make you feel better. No one, not even a doctor or nutritionist, can really save you if you are not willing to work hard on improving your lifestyle. What we put inside of our bodies every day has major consequences.

Human health is just as important as history or long division, is it not? Everyone should know the basics as early as possible. Yet nutrition is not a priority in most elementary or middle schools. Without this knowledge, how can we really understand weight loss? Educate yourself and stay current on new research about nutrition by focusing on the facts. Use credible sources such as scientific journals, credentialed experts in nutrition, and books with diverse scientific references. Build a support team of health-conscious individuals and make your goals a reality!

If we have the power to prevent deadly chronic diseases, then why not take advantage of that power? Start by taking the fourteen-day challenge at the end of this book. Or if you refuse to eat even one meal without meat, start by making small changes toward a diet based mostly on natural plant foods. If the thought of changing your entire diet is too overwhelming, start with a "Meatless Monday." Taste a different food every week, whether it is a Thai vegetable curry, an Indian chana masala dish, or a Mexican mushroom fajita dish. One way to track improvement is by choosing a realistic goal, such as eat one whole fruit and something green every day. Then increase this goal to two fruits and two cups of veggies daily. Continue to progress with your goals each month until most of your diet is made up of healthy plant foods. Try the fourteen-day challenge in the next chapter with a friend or family member.

During the average workweek, I see people at the end stages of life, and most are suffering a terrible fate of the American diet. The patients have a history of obesity, high cholesterol, hypertension, dementia, heart failure and the list goes on. Yet this fate is not inevitable. I see many people make small changes every day that can have profound impacts on their health. It is certainly not impossible. Think of your future and your family's future. Make a commitment to your health and longevity today.

Links

Check out free health tips: fitwithjen.com
Like my page: facebook.com/fitwjen
Enjoy free recipes: pinterest.com/fitwithjen7
Follow me on Twitter: fitwithjencom

Tips for Die-Hard Meat Eaters

- Count your fiber grams.
- Add beans to your salads, soups, and entrees.
- Aim for a minimum 30–40 g of fiber a day.
- Plan your meals around vegetables instead of meat.
- Eat a source of omega-3 daily; for example, chia seeds, flaxseeds, or sustainable fish.
- Taste different meat substitutes like veggie burgers, soy "chicken," or faux deli slices.
- Avoid processed or red meat, as these are high in AGEs, heterocyclic amines, and/or heme iron.
- Keep a close eye on your cholesterol, blood pressure, and inflammation (Hs CRP/ESR).

Tips for Aspiring Vegetarians/Vegans

- Try new recipes with beans, greens, nuts, and seeds.
- Aim for a minimum of 40 g of fiber daily.
- Try favorite recipes using meat and dairy substitutes.
- Find ways to include seaweed or veggie sushi in meals.
- Keep an eye on your iron and vitamin D levels via blood tests.
- Take small steps instead of making a huge lifestyle change.
- Don't feel guilty if you fall off the wagon once in a while.

Tips for Long-Time Vegans

- Add lemon juice or another source of vitamin C to meals to increase mineral absorption.
- Cook with cast-iron pans and lemon or lime juice to raise iron content of meals and to increase iron absorption.
- Aim for an average of 50 g of fiber daily.
- Find a vegan source of the essential omega-3 fat DHA.
- Make sure to get iodine via sea vegetables or veggie sushi.

- Test your vitamin B_{12}, vitamin D, ferritin (iron stores), and homocysteine yearly.
- Take a supplement when vitamin or mineral levels are low.

FAQs on How Plant Eaters Can Avoid Nutrient Deficiency

- **Should vegans limit salt intake?** No, the average vegan has low blood pressure,[18, 19] so there's no need to be scared of salty foods, especially since faux sausage is much lower in sodium than real sausage. The recommendations offered in this book ensure that enough potassium, which can lower blood pressure, is included in the diet. But just to stay on the safe side, check blood pressure once a month. If it's high, make sure to eat more potassium-rich foods like baked potatoes, mushrooms, dry fruit, and beans.
- **Are vegans at risk of osteoporosis because they eat less calcium?** Not necessarily. Vegans do not have significantly different rates of osteoporosis than do meat eaters.[20–22] In fact, consuming high amounts of animal products and corticosteroids is more likely to result in bone loss.[21] Bone density is affected by weight, so obese people often have higher bone density when compared with normal weight people. The most important thing you can do to protect your bones is to lift weights, especially for those above the age of 65, and eat plenty of green vegetables. Progressive strength exercises (not high-rep exercises) that gradually increase weight/ resistance (low reps) over time can help. Some of the best exercises to work up to are lunges, squats, pull-ups, push-ups, and dips. This is crucial for vegans who are skinny and usually stay that way as seniors.
- **How do you get calcium on a vegan diet?** Green, leafy veggies like kale and broccoli have plenty of calcium, so they should be eaten daily. Beans, tofu, and fortified nondairy milk also contain calcium.
- **Who needs vitamin D supplements?** Everyone who does not get 75% of his or her skin exposed to the sun for a minimum of

fifteen minutes daily could benefit from vitamin D supplements. Vitamin D deficiency is becoming increasingly common for meat eaters and vegans alike, because humans, on the whole, no longer work or exercise outdoors. Check your vitamin D status through a blood test every year. If it's low, then take a vitamin D supplement and recheck it each year.

- **Do vegetarians more often have iron deficiency than meat eaters?** Vegetarians do not have iron deficiency more often than do meat eaters.[23] In fact, vegans and vegetarians eat more iron than meat eaters do, but vegans may be at a risk for deficiency, because of phytates and oxalates.[17, 23, 24] This is not, however, an excuse to indulge in a daily dose of beef for obtaining heme iron. For every milligram of meat-based iron consumed, there is an increase in risk of cancer, which does not occur with supplemental or plant-based iron.[25–27] Meat eaters have double the iron stores when compared with vegetarians.[24] This is likely why meat eaters have a higher risk of cancer and diabetes, along with the fact that they are heavier than vegetarians on average. Phytates and oxalates in beans, grains, and vegetables protect the body from storing dangerous levels of iron. When iron stores decrease below normal, the body adapts to absorb more iron from plant foods and supplements.[28, 29] When iron stores are high, however, the body cannot adapt to absorb less iron from meat.[28, 29] So a healthy way to improve iron status is to prepare beans, vegetables, and grains with lemon or lime juice in cast-iron cookware.[30–32] After a few months, eating food regularly cooked in iron pots can even increase hemoglobin levels.[32]

- **Which vegan foods are high in iron?** White beans and kidney beans are rich in iron with about double the amount that's in a 9-oz sirloin steak.[33] However, drinking coffee or tea with a meal is detrimental, because coffee and tea both block the absorption of iron.[34] Orange juice or lemonade with meals would be a much better choice for people with anemia.

- **Do vegans have vitamin B_{12} deficiency?** According to some studies, about 50% of vegans have vitamin B_{12} deficiency, because they often do not take supplements or eat sufficiently fortified food.[35, 36] This is a vitamin made by bacteria found naturally in the soil and on dirty vegetables. Since modern humans wash and cook their food, plants are no longer a good source of B_{12}. Animals store the vitamin in their flesh after eating "dirty" plant foods. If you are 100% vegan, then you should check your B_{12} levels each year and take a supplement before becoming deficient. Some breakfast cereals and nondairy milks are fortified with B_{12}.

- **How do I get enough omega-3 fat?** Flaxseeds and chia seeds are high in an omega-3 fat known as ALA. Humans need three different types of omega-3 fat for brain and heart health: ALA, EPA, and DHA. The body converts a decent amount of ALA into EPA, but it does not convert enough ALA to DHA to meet its needs.[37] The best source of DHA is microalgae, so vegetarians and omnivores who do not eat fish can take a supplement to ensure an adequate intake.[37]

Notes

1. Tonstad S, Butler T, Yan R, Fraser GE. "Type of vegetarian diet, body weight, and prevalence of type 2 diabetes." *Diabetes Care* 2009; 32 (5): 791-6.
2. Zhang HJ, Han P, Sun SY, Wang LY, Yan B, Zhang JH, et al. "Attenuated associations between increasing BMI and unfavorable lipid profiles in Chinese Buddhist vegetarians." *Asia Pac J Clin* 2013; 22 (2): 249-56.
3. Peterson BJ, Anoushan R, Fan J, Jaceldo-Siegl K, Fraser GE. "Vegetarian diets and blood pressure among white subjects from the Adventist Health Study 2 (AHS-2)." *Public Health Nutr* 2012; 15 (10): 1909-1916.
4. Bradbury KE, Crowe FL, Appleby PN, Schmidt JA, Travis RC, Key TJ. "Serum concentration of cholesterol, apolipoprotein A-I and apolipoprotein B in a total of 1694 meat-eaters, fish-eaters, vegetarians and vegans." *Eur J Clin Nutr* 2014; 68 (2): 178-83.

5. Kim MK, Cho SW, Park YK. "Long-term vegetarians have low oxidative stress, body fat, and cholesterol levels." *Nutr Res Pract* 2012; 6 (2): 155-61.

6. Ambroszkiewicz J, Klemarczyk W, Gajewska J, Chelchowska M, Rowicka G, Oltarzewski M, et al. "Serum concentration of adipocytokines in prepubertal vegetarian and omnivorous children." *Med Wieku Rozwoj* 2011; 15 (3): 326-34.

7. Vinagre JC, Vinagre CG, Pozzi FS, Slywitch E, Maranhao RC. "Metabolism of triglyceride-rich lipoproteins and transfer of lipids to high-density lipoproteins (HDL) in vegan and omnivore subjects." *Nutr Metab Cardiovasc Dis* 2013; 23 (1): 61-7.

8. Sutliffe JT, Wilson LD, de Heer HD, Foster RL, Carnot MJ. "C-reactive protein response to a vegan lifestyle intervention." *Complement Ther Med* 2015; 23 (1): 32-7.

9. Pettersen BJ, Anousheh R, Fan J, Jaceldo-Siegl K, Fraser GE. "Vegetarian diets and blood pressure among white subjects: results from the Adventist Health Study 2 (AHS-2)." *Public Health Nutr* 2012; 15 (10): 1909-1916.

10. "High Cholesterol Facts", Centers for Disease Control and Prevention, Accessed September 5, 2015, http://www.cdc.gov/cholesterol/facts.htm.

11. Carroll MD, Lacher DA, Sorlie PD, Cleeman JI, Gordon DJ, Wolz M, et al. "Trends in serum lipids and lipoproteins of adults", 1960-2002. *JAMA* 2005; 294 (14): 1773-81.

12. Ong KL, Allison MA, Cheung BM, Wu BJ, Barter PJ, Rye KA. "Trends in C-reactive protein levels in the US adults from 1999 to 2010." *Am J Epidemiol* 2013; 177 (12): 1430-42.

13. Zhang HJ, Han P, Sun SY, Wang LY, Yan B, Zhang JH, et al. "Attenuated associations between increasing BMI and unfavorable lipid profiles in Chinese Buddhist vegetarians." *Asia Pac J Clin* 2013; 22 (2): 249-256.

14. Thorogood M, Carter R, Benfield L, McPherson K, Mann JI. "Plasma lipids and lipoprotein cholesterol concentrations in people with different diets in Britain." *Br Med J (Clin Res Ed)* 1987; 295 (6594): 351-353.

15. Waldmann A, Koschizke JW, Leitzmann C, Hahn A. "German vegan study: diet, life-style factors, and cardiovascular risk profile." *Ann Nutr Metab* 2005; 49 (6): 366-72.

16. See Appendix A.

17. Clarys P, Deliens T, Huybrechts I, Deiremaeker P, Vanaelst B, De Keyzer W, et al. "Comparison of nutritional quality of the vegan, vegetarian, semi-vegetairan, pesco-vegetarian and omnivorous diet." *Nutrients* 2014; 6 (3): 1318-32.

18. Fraser GE, Shavlik DJ. "Risk factors for all-cause and coronary heart disease mortality in the oldest-old." The Adventist Health Study. *Arch Intern Med* 1997; 157 (19): 2249-58.

19. Martinez-Gonzalez MA, Sanchez-Tainta A, Corella D, Salas-Salvado J, Ros E, Aros F, et al. "A provegetarian food pattern and re-duction in total mortality in the Prevencion con Dieta Mediterranea (PREDIMED) study." *Am J Clin Nutr* 2014; 100 (s1): 320s-328s.

20. Ho-Pham LT, Nguyen PL, Le TT, Doan TA, Tran NT, Le Ta, et al. "Veganism, bone mineral density, and body composition: a study in Buddhist nuns." *Osteoporsosis Int* 2009; 20 (12): 2087-93.

21. Ho-Pham LT, Vu BQ, Lai TQ, Nguyen ND, Nguyen TV. "Vegetarianism, bone loss, fracture and vitamin D: a longitudinal study in Asian vegans and non-vegans." *Eur J Clin Nutr* 2012; 66 (1): 75-82.

22. Wang YF, Chiu JS, Chuang MH, Chiu JE, Lin CL. "Bone mineral density of vegetarian and non-vegetarian adults in Taiwan." *Asia Pac J Clin Nutr* 2008; 17 (1): 101-6.

23. Craig WJ. "Iron status of vegetarians." *Am J Clin Nutr* 1994; 59 (5 suppl): 1233s-1237.

24. Shaw NS, Chin CJ, Pan WH. "A vegetarian diet rich in soybean products compromises iron status in young students." *J Nutr* 1995; 125 (2): 212-9.

25. Fonseca-Nunez A, Jakszyn P, Agudo A. "Iron and cancer risk-a sys-tematic review and meta-analysis of the epidemiological evidence." *Cancer Epidemiol Biomarkers Prev* 2014; 23(1): 12-31.

26. Qiao L, Fung Y. "Intakes of heme iron and zinc and colorectal cancer incidence: a meta-analysis of prospective studies." *Cancer Causes Control* 2013; 24 (6): 1175-83.

27. Baharvand M, Manifar S, Akkafan R, Mortazavi H, Sabour S. "Serum levels of ferritin, copper, and zinc in patients with oral cancer." *Biomed J* 2014; 37 (5): 331-6.

28. Hunt JR, Roughead ZK. "Adaptation of iron absorption in men consuming diets with high or low iron bioavailability." *Am J Clin Nutr* 2000; 71 (1): 94-102.

29. Roughead ZK, Hunt JR. "Adaptation in iron absorption: iron supplementation reduces nonheme-iron but not heme-iron absorption from food." *Am J Clin Nutr* 2000: 72 (4): 982-9.

30. Charles CV, Summerlee AJ, Dewey CE. "Iron content of Cambodian foods when prepared in cooking pots containing an iron ingot." *Trop Med Int Health* 2011;16 (12): 1518-24.

31. Prinsen Geerligs PD, Brabin BJ, Hart DJ, Fairweather-Tait SJ. "Iron contents of Malawian foods when prepared in iron cooking pots." *Int J Vitam Nutr Res* 2004; 74 (1): 21-6.

32. Kulkami SA, Ekbote VH, Sonawane A, Jevakumar A, Chiplonkar SA, Khadilkar AV. "Beneficial effect of iron pot cooking on iron status." *Indian J Pediatr* 2013; 80 (12): 985-9.

33. U.S. Department of Agriculture, Agricultural Research Service. 2014. USDA National Nutrient Database for Standard Reference, Release 27. Nutrient Data Laboratory Home Page, Accessed February 25, 2015, http://www.ars.usda.gov/nutrientdata.

34. Morck TA, Lynch SR, Cook JD. "Inhibition of food iron absorption by coffee." *Am J Clin Nutr* 1983; 37 (3): 416-20.

35. Pawlak R, Lester SE, Babatunde T. "The prevalence of cobalamin deficiency among vegetarians assessed by serum vitamin B12: a review of literature." *Eur J Clin Nutr* 2014; 68 (5): 541-8.

36. Gilsing AM, Crowe FL, Lloyd-Wright Z, Sanders TA, Appleby PN, Allen NE, Key TJ. "Serum concentrations of vitamin B12 and folate in British male omnivores, vegetarians and vegans: results from a cross-sectional analysis of the EPIC-Oxford cohort study." *Eur J Clin Nutr* 2010; 64 (9): 933-9.

37. Lane K, Derbyshire E, Li W, Brennan C. "Bioavailability and potential uses of vegetarian sources of omega-3 fatty acids: a review of the literature." *Crit Rev Food Sci Nutr* 2014; 54 (5): 572-9.

CHAPTER 12

Fourteen-Day
Challenge Meal Plan

Think you are ready to try a plant-based lifestyle? Try this fourteen-day meat-free challenge to see how easy or hard it is giving up animal products. The following meals are exclusively made from plants with an emphasis on whole foods. They include some processed food, such as tofu and dairy-free cheese, to make meals fast and convenient. If you are willing to spend more time making homemade cashew cheese and meat substitutes instead of buying pre-packaged dairy-free cheese or faux meats then more power to you! Mock meats are usually lower in fat and cholesterol compared to real meats. The recipes are in no particular order and can be switch up for convenience.

Save the long recipes for weekends if necessary. Double or triple these recipes to have plenty of leftovers that can be frozen or refrigerated for several days after they are made. I share some of my favorite recipes in this section and most are at least centered on whole foods. But when time is limited I occasionally warm up a frozen veggie burger, dog, or use dairy-free cheese substitutes to dress up salads and make simple meals with adequate protein. You can eat a plant-based diet without these processed foods, however, it may take more effort and time to make veggie and whole grain recipes taste good. For those who like or miss the taste and feel of meat, there are many new and improved substitutes available.

The meal plan is a balanced mix of foods to satisfy different tastes. Make sure to do some grocery shopping with a list of items from this book so your kitchen is ready too. Some of the ingredients such as chia seeds and nutritional yeast are easier to find in a health food store or online instead of a regular grocery store.

Kitchen essentials:

- Agave
- Almond Milk
- Chia seeds
- Extra Firm Tofu
- Nutritional yeast
- Tempeh
- Vegan Butter
- Vegan Mayo
- Vegan Cheese

This meal plan is made for a woman of average height who needs 1400-1600 calories daily depending on physical activity level. Most women need 50-60 grams of protein daily unless they are athletes. For men or very active women, the same meal plan with a double serving of dinner can suffice with a total of 1900-2000 daily calories. Eating two servings of the dinner meal can also bring the protein total closer to 70 grams, which is sufficient to meet protein needs for the average man. Each person has different needs so it is important to monitor weight/body composition and adjust calories accordingly. (The calories and protein are rough estimates in each meal and may vary in practice.)

Time to Eat!

14 Day Meal Plan Day 1	
Day 1 **Breakfast** *Cocoa Peanut Butter Shake* Time: 5 min Serves 1 Calories: 432 Protein: 14 g	Ingredients: 1 c almond milk original 1 banana 1 T chia seeds 1 T cocoa powder 2 T natural peanut butter (stir it and keep refrigerated to avoid separation) Directions: Place all ingredients in a high-speed blender like a Nutribullet or Vita Mix and blend until smooth. Add a few cubes of ice if necessary to keep cool.
Day 1 **Snack** Calories: 176 Protein: 5 g	Ingredients: 1 c cherries ½ oz pistachios Directions: Rinse and serve fruit with nuts.
Day 1 **Lunch** *Black Bean Avocado Salad* Time: 20 min Serves 4 Calories: 440 Protein: 14 g	Ingredients: 1 avocado, sliced 2 cans of black beans, Rinsed 2 ears of corn, scraped from the cob 2 carrots, chopped 8 grape tomatoes ¼ c purple onion, finely chopped ½ c red bell pepper, chopped ¼ c parsley, chopped 2 garlic cloves, minced

	¼ c canola oil salt to taste Directions: Mix all ingredients except the garlic and oil together. Whisk garlic and oil in a separate bowl until well blended. Pour the garlic oil over the rest of the ingredients and serve.
Day 1 **Dinner** ***Coconut Curry Chickpeas*** Time: 2 hours Serves 5 Calories: 480 Protein: 22 g **Total calories: 1528** **Total protein: 55 g**	Ingredients: 1 bag of chickpeas, pre-cooked 1 c onion, finely chopped 4 cloves garlic, minced 1 can coconut milk 2 cans of diced tomatoes 2 carrots 2 c brown rice 1 T curry powder 1 tsp salt ½ tsp crushed red pepper ½ c cilantro, chopped Directions: Cook rice according to package directions. Heat oil in a Dutch oven or regular large pot over medium heat; add onion and garlic, and cook 5 minutes. Add chickpeas, tomatoes, coconut milk, curry powder, salt and crushed red pepper. Cover, reduce heat, cook 15 minutes. Uncover, and cook 10 minutes longer. Stir in cilantro, and serve over cooked brown rice.

Day 2	
Day 2 **Breakfast** ***Strawberry Oatmeal*** Time: 5 minutes Serves 1 Calories: 329 Protein: 7 g	<u>Ingredients:</u> ½ c oats, old fashioned ½ c strawberries, diced 1 c almond milk, original 1 T agave (optional for the 'sweet tooth') 1 T walnuts, chopped <u>Directions:</u> Pour milk, agave and oats into a sauce pan over medium heat for 6 minutes. Add strawberries and serve in a bowl.
Day 2 **Snack** Calories: 248 Protein: 7 g	<u>Ingredients:</u> 1 c blueberries 1 oz almonds <u>Directions:</u> Rinse and serve fruit with nuts.
Day 2 **Lunch** ***Black Bean Avocado Salad*** Time: 5 minutes Serves 1 Calories: 260 Protein: 6 g	Use one serving of the leftovers from day 1 lunch.

Day 2 **Dinner** *Coconut Curry Chickpeas* Time: 5 minutes Serves 1 Calories: 480 Protein: 22 g **Total calories: 1497** **Total protein: 49 g**	Use leftovers from day 1 dinner.
Day 3	
Day 3 **Breakfast** *Tofu Scramble* Time: 20 minutes Serves 2 (double for leftovers) Calories: 222 Protein: 23 g	Ingredients: 1 package of tofu ½ bell pepper, diced 1 c onion, diced 1 T garlic powder 3 T nutritional yeast 1 T soy sauce Salt to taste Directions: Heat oil in a large pan then add onion and bell pepper. Cook for 4 minutes on medium heat. Add crumbled tofu and all the other ingredients. Cook until all the liquid is gone then serve.
Day 3 **Snack** Calories: 263 Protein: 5 g	Ingredients: 1 large peach 1 oz pecans Directions: Rinse and serve fruit with nuts.

Day 3 **Lunch** *Mock Tuna Sandwich* Time: 20 minutes Serves 5 Calories: 302 Protein: 18 g	Mock Tuna Ingredients: 1 8oz pack of tempeh, chopped 2 celery stalks 2 T onion, finely chopped 1/3 c vegan mayo, (I use Vegenaise) 1 T vinegar 1 T seaweed flakes Sandwich Ingredients: 2 sl whole wheat toast ½ cup raw spinach Directions: Cover tempeh with water and simmer in a pot for 20 min. Remove from heat and drain the excess liquid. Add the remaining tuna ingredients and mix well. Place the mock tuna and spinach in between the two slices of toast, cut in half and serve.
Day 3 **Dinner** *Miso Mushroom Soup* Time: 5 minutes Serves 1 Calories: 334 Protein: 22 g **Total calories: 1425** **Total protein: 68 g**	Ingredients: 1 package of mushrooms 4 t miso 1 pack of tofu, cubed 5 c vegetable broth 2 t seaweed 1 scallion, chopped 1 c brown rice, cooked Directions: Add all ingredients to a pot, bring to a boil, then simmer for 25 minutes. Serve hot.

Day 4	
Day 4 **Breakfast** ***Tofu Scramble leftovers*** Time: 5 minutes Serves 2 Calories: 222 Protein: 23 g	Use leftovers from day 3 breakfast.
Day 4 **Snack** Calories: 326 Protein: 8 g	Ingredients: 1 apple 2 T natural peanut butter Directions: Rinse apple and cut into slices. Dip slices in peanut butter.
Day 4 **Lunch** ***Crunchy Cashew Rainbow Salad*** Time: 20 minutes Serves 5 Calories: 358 Protein: 7 g	Ingredients: 1 head of bok choy, chopped 1 red bell pepper, diced 2 carrots, diced ½ c canola oil ¼ c cider vinegar ½ c cashews ¼ c cashews, chopped (garnish) 2 T brown sugar ½ t salt Directions: Add oil, vinegar, peanuts, and brown sugar to the blender and process until smooth. Combine bok choy, bell pepper, and carrots in a bowl, mix well and serve.

Day 4 Dinner ***Stuffed Sweet Potato*** Time: 20 minutes Serves 3 Calories: 487 Protein: 12 g **Total calories: 1393** **Total protein: 50 g**	Ingredients: 4 sweet potatoes 1 10oz pack of raw spinach 1 T onion powder 5 T vegan butter (I use Earth Balance) ½ c chopped scallions ½ c peanuts, crushed Directions: Preheat oven to 450 degrees. Place sweet potatoes directly on oven rack. Cook them for 40 minutes. Cut cooked sweet potatoes in half and scrape the insides, then combine this with spinach, onion powder, scallions and butter in a separate bowl. Refill the potato skins up with equal amounts of the mixture in each skin. Place back in the oven on a baking sheet for 10 minutes, sprinkle with peanuts then serve.
Day 5	
Day 5 **Breakfast** ***Kale Flax Shake*** Time: 5 minutes Serves 1 Calories: 288 Protein: 8 g	Ingredients: 1 c almond milk unsweet or original 1 banana ½ c strawberries 2 T flax seeds 1 c kale leaves, (stems removed) Directions: Place all ingredients in a high-speed blender like a Nutribullet or Vita Mix and blend until smooth. Add a few cubes of ice if necessary to keep cool.

Day 5 Snack Calories: 268 Protein: 5 g	Ingredients: 1 c grapes ¼ c walnuts Directions: Rinse and serve.
Day 5 Lunch ***Eggless Salad Sandwich*** Time: 10 min Serves 6 Calories: 361 Protein: 25 g	Ingredients: 16 oz tofu block, crumbled 2 dill pickles minced 5 celery sticks, chopped 1 garlic clove, minced ½ cup vegan mayo (I use Follow Your Heart brand) 2 T dijon mustard 2 T nutritional yeast 1 T soy sauce or tamari 1 t turmeric 1 t curry powder salt to taste 12 sl whole wheat bread Directions: Mix all ingredients except for tofu in a bowl and whisk for 1 minute. Add crumbled tofu, mix well and serve in between two slices of bread.
Day 5 Dinner ***Garlic Mushroom Spaghetti*** Time: 10 min Serves 3 Calories: 436 Protein: 15 g **Total calories: 1353**	Ingredients: 2 8oz packs of sliced mushrooms 5 garlic cloves, minced ¼ c olives 1 c artichoke hearts 1 jar spaghetti sauce (choose dairy-free) 1 onion, diced 1 shallot 1 pack whole wheat spaghetti

Total protein: 53 g	2 T canola oil salt to taste Directions: Heat oil in a Dutch oven or regular large pot over medium heat; add onion, shallot, mushrooms and garlic, and cook 5 minutes. Add tomato sauce to mix and cook extra 5 minutes. Cook spaghetti according to package directions, drain, then stir in mushroom mix and serve.
Day 6	
Day 6 **Breakfast** ***Peaches 'n' Cream Style Bagel*** Time: 10 min Serves 1 Calories: 367 Protein: 10 g	Ingredients: 1 whole wheat bagel, toasted 2 ½ T vegan cream cheese (I use Go Veggie brand) 1 peach, sliced ¼ c almonds, sliced Directions: Add peaches and vegan cream cheese to a bowl. Use a fork to mash the peaches and mix with the cream cheese. Spread this mix on the bagel, top with almonds and serve.
Day 6 **Snack** Calories: 157 Protein: 8 g	Ingredients: 1 c chopped pineapple 1 c soy milk Directions: Core, skin, chop and serve (or choose pre-chopped fruit).

| **Day 6**
Lunch

Lemon Garlic Quinoa
Time: 10 min
Serves 3
Calories: 489
Protein: 16.5 g | Ingredients:
2 T organic canola oil
4 c quinoa
4 c vegetable broth
2 c green peas (may be from frozen)
1 lemon
4 cloves garlic, minced
1 onion, finely diced
Salt to taste

Directions:
Cook garlic, oil, and onion over medium heat for 5 minutes. Cook quinoa in a separate pot with veggie broth for 30 minutes, then add garlic mix, sprinkle with lemon juice, salt, and serve. |
| **Day 6**
Dinner

Veggie Chili Beans
Time: 10 min
Serves 4
Calories: 400
Protein: 22 g
Total calories: 1413
Total protein: 56.5 g | Ingredients:
2 T organic canola oil
1 c onion, chopped
2 T garlic, minced
1 jalapeno, finely chopped
1 zucchini, diced
1 c carrots, diced
2 packs of mushrooms, chopped
2 T chili powder
1 T cumin
1 t salt
2 T garlic powder
1 T onion powder
¼ t cayenne pepper
4 large tomatoes, chopped
3 c cooked kidney beans
1 15 oz can tomato sauce
½ c cilantro, chopped |

	Directions: Heat oil in a large pot over medium heat and add onions, bell peppers, garlic and jalapeno. Cook for 5 minutes then add all the veggies for additional 5 minutes. Add all of the other ingredients and cook for 20 minutes then serve.
Day 7	
Day 7 **Breakfast** *Green Chia Protein Shake* Time: 5 minutes Serves 1 Calories: 429 Protein: 14 g	Ingredients: 1 c original almond milk 1 banana 2 T peanut 1 T chia seeds 1 c spinach 1 t vanilla extract Directions: Put all ingredients in a blender or Vita Mix and blend until smooth.
Day 7 **Snack** Calories: 281 Protein: 7 g	Ingredients: 1 pear 1 soy yogurt Directions: Rinse, slice and serve.
Day 7 **Lunch** *Mock Chicken Salad Sandwich* Time: 10 min Serves 4 Calories: 352 Protein: 29 g	Ingredients: 1 tomato, sliced 1 c raw spinach 2 slices whole grain bread, toasted 2 c chopped vegan chicken (I use 1 pack Gardein chick'n scallopini, (480 kcal) 1/3 c vegan mayo (I prefer Vegenaise) ½ lemon

	1T mustard 2 scallions 1 tsp fresh dill 2 stalks celery, chopped ½ tsp salt Directions: Sauté chick'n 6-10 min until golden. Chop and mix all other ingredients in a mixer then combine with chick'n, stir and serve.
Day 7 **Dinner** *Veggie Chili Leftovers* Time: 5 min Serves 2 Calories: 400 Protein: 22 g **Total calories: 1462** **Total protein: 72 g**	Ingredients: 2 c veggie chili leftovers 2 c brown rice, cooked Directions: Warm up chili and rice then serve.
Day 8	
Day 8 **Breakfast** *Cinnamon Vegan French Toast* Time: 10 min Serves 2 Calories: 461 Protein: 14 g	Ingredients: 6 slices whole wheat bread, toasted 2 c almond milk original 1.5 T flax meal (ground flax seeds) 1 T maple syrup 2 T vegan butter 1 t vanilla extract 1 t cinnamon Directions: Whisk together almond milk, flax, vanilla and cinnamon in a bowl and place

	in freezer for 15 minutes. Cut toast in four slices each to resemble French toast sticks. Dip sticks in batter then cook in a pan over medium-high heat with a small portion of vegan butter for each batch. Cook until each slice is golden brown then serve with fresh berries or additional maple syrup.
Day 8 **Snack** Calories: 170 Protein: 6.5 g	Ingredients: 1 orange 2 T pumpkin or sunflower seeds Directions: Rinse and serve.
Day 8 **Lunch** *Whole Grain Pasta Salad* Time: 10 min Serves 3 Calories: 283 Protein: 13 g	Ingredients: 2 c whole grain macaroni, cooked 1 c tomato, chopped ½ c celery, chopped ¼ c red onion, finely diced ½ c vegan mayo (I use Vegenaise) ½ t agave 3 T nutritional yeast 1 T mustard 1 T cider vinegar 1 t black pepper ½ t salt Directions: Mix the last seven ingredients together in a bowl. Then pour this mixture over cooked macaroni and combine with the remaining ingredients. (Save leftovers) Stir everything for a few seconds then serve.

Day 8 Dinner *Cabbage Soup* Time: 45 min Serves 3 Calories: 546 Protein: 23 g **Total calories: 1460** **Total protein: 56.5 g**	Ingredients: 6 slices whole grain toast 2 T organic canola oil 6 c green cabbage, chopped 1 onion, diced 4 c vegetable broth 1(15oz) jar or can of plain tomato sauce 2 T nutritional yeast ½ t coriander seeds ½ t cumin 1 t black pepper ½ t salt Directions: Heat oil in a large pot and add onion. Cook for 5 minutes then add all of the other ingredients and cook for 35 minutes then serve.
	Day 9
Day 9 **Breakfast** *Raisin Bran & Blueberries* Time: 5 min Serves 1 Calories: 458 Protein: 19.5 g	Ingredients: 1 c raisin bran (I use organic store brand) 1 c soy milk ¼ c fresh blueberries ¼ c raw almonds, chopped Directions: Mix all ingredients in a bowl and serve.
Day 9 **Snack** Calories: 288 Protein: 7.5 g	Ingredients: 1 small apple 2 T peanut butter Directions: Rinse and serve.

| Day 9 Lunch

Grilled Vegan Cheese Sandwich
Time: 10 min
Serves 1
Calories: 517
Protein: 10 g | Ingredients:
2 slices whole grain toast
2 slices of vegan cheese (I use Chao cheese by Field Roast)
2 T vegan butter (I use Earth Balance brand)
1 slice of onion

Directions:
Heat oil then add the slice of onion and cooked for 3-5 minutes until is started to brown. Spread vegan butter on both sides of each slice of bread. Place the vegan cheese in between the slices of bread and cook on a separate pan over medium heat for 1 minute. Turn the sandwich over until each side is cooked for 1 to 1.5 minutes. Open the cooked sandwich, add the slice of onion, close, cut in half and serve. |
| Day 9 Dinner

Veggie Fried Rice
Time: 10 min
Serves 3
Calories: 395
Protein: 17 g
Total calories: 1650
Total protein: 54 g | Ingredients:
4 c brown rice, cooked
2 c onions, diced
3 c mushrooms, cubed
2 c peas, frozen
½ c scallions, chopped
½ c green bell pepper, chopped
3 cloves of garlic, minced
2 T soy sauce
1 T sesame oil
½ t salt

Directions:
Heat oil in a dutch oven before adding onion, garlic, and bell pepper. Cook |

	for 5 minutes then add all the other ingredients, stir, and continue cooking for 10 minutes then serve.
Day 10	
Day 10 **Breakfast** *Green Chia Shake* Time: 5 min Serves 1 Calories: 524 Protein: 23.2 g	Ingredients: 1 c soy milk 1 banana 2 T almond butter 2 T chia seeds 1 c spinach 1 t vanilla extract Directions: Put all ingredients in a blender or Vita Mix and blend until smooth.
Day 10 **Snack** Calories: 209 Protein: 7 g	Ingredients: 1 c strawberries 1 oz. almonds Directions: Rinse and serve.
Day 10 **Lunch** *Pasta Salad Leftovers* Time: 10 min Serves 1 Calories: 283 Protein: 15 g	Use the leftover pasta salad from day 8, add 2 T toasted sunflower seeds and enjoy.

Day 10 Dinner *Baked Lemon Veggies* Time: 10 min Serves 3 Calories: 368 Protein: 22 g **Total calories: 1384** **Total protein: 67.2 g**	Ingredients: 2 c mushrooms 2 c zucchini, diced 1 onion, finely chopped 2 c red bell pepper 2 c quinoa, cooked in veggie broth 2 c edamame 4 vegan sausages (I use Tofurkey apple) 2 T garlic powder 1 lemon ½ t salt Directions: Preheat oven to 400 degrees. Place all veggies and edamame in a large casserole dish then cover with lemon juice, garlic powder
Day 11	
Day 11 Breakfast *Green Chia Shake* Time: 10 min Serves 6 Calories: 426 Protein: 14 g	Ingredients: 1 c original almond milk 1 banana 2 T peanut 1 T chia seeds 1 c spinach 1 t vanilla extract Directions: Put all ingredients in a blender or Vita Mix and blend until smooth

Day 11 **Snack** Calories: 83 Protein: 1 g	Ingredients: ½ c dried figs Directions: Halve and serve.
Day 11 **Lunch** ***Zucchini Peanut Pasta*** Time: 10 min Serves 2 Calories: 321 Protein: 15 g	Ingredients: 4 whole zucchini 2 carrots, grated ¼ c peanut butter 1 T soy sauce 1 T lime juice 1 t agave 2 T basil, chopped Pinch of crushed red pepper Salt to taste Directions: Use a Veggetti or similar tool to shred zucchini into a thin pasta-like texture. Combine carrots with zucchini in one bowl. Mix all other ingredients in a separate bowl. Pour the seasoning mix onto the zucchini bowl, stir and serve.
Day 11 **Dinner** ***Savory Chick'n Lettuce Wraps*** Time: 5 min Serves 6 Calories: 436 Protein: 36 g **Total calories: 1266** **Total protein: 66 g**	Ingredients: 3 c black-eyed peas 1 bag frozen corn 2 tomatoes 1 c mock chicken, diced (I use Beyond Meat brand) 2 T oil 3 T nutritional yeast 2 shallots, thinly sliced 3 garlic cloves, minced 1 lemon, quartered 12 romaine lettuce leaves

	Directions: Heat oil in a pan over medium heat, then add shallots and garlic. Cook for 2 minutes then add corn and cook for 6 more minutes. Combine corn mix with all other ingredients, sprinkle lemon juice over them evenly and serve.
Day 12	
Day 12 **Breakfast** ***Blueberry Coconut Parfait*** Time: 10 min Serves 1 Calories: 511 Protein: 9 g	Ingredients: ½ c blueberries ¼ c coconut flakes ¼ c pecans, chopped ¼ c granola (several types are dairy free, just read the ingredients label) 1 T chia seeds 1 vanilla flavored coconut yogurt Directions: Using a tall glass jar or mug, layer the berries, coconut, nuts, yogurt and granola then serve.
Day 12 **Snack** Calories: 152 Protein: 9.5 g	Ingredients: 1 c raspberries 1 c soy milk Directions: Rinse and serve.
Day 12 **Lunch** ***Spicy Hummus Sandwich*** Time: 10 min Serves 1	Ingredients: ½ c hummus (Sabra brand is tasty!) 2 slices of tomato 2 slices of lettuce 2 slices of whole grain bread 1 t hot sauce

Calories: 459 Protein: 17 g	Directions: Toast bread if desired. Spread hummus on one side of bread and add other ingredients then close sandwich, cut in half and serve.
Day 12 **Dinner** *Garlic Cauliflower Mash* Time: 10 min Serves 3 Calories: 370 Protein: 25 g **Total calories: 1492** **Total protein: 61 g**	Ingredients: 1 head of cauliflower, steamed 2 T vegan butter 1 T garlic powder ½ c vegan cheese (I use mozzarella style Daiya) 2 T nutritional yeast 1 package of beefless tips (I use Gardein) 1 lemon 1 T organic canola oil Directions: Steam cauliflower with garlic powder. Place all ingredients except faux meat in a food processor and process until creamy. Cook beefless tips according to package directions and add lemon juice while cooking. (Save leftovers) Serve with cauliflower mash.
Day 13	
Day 13 **Breakfast** *Raspberry Coconut Parfait* Time: 10 min Serves 1 Calories: 609 Protein: 10 g	Ingredients: ½ c raspberries ¼ c coconut flakes ¼ c walnuts, chopped ¼ c granola (several types are dairy free) 1 vanilla flavored coconut yogurt

	Directions: Using a tall glass jar or mug, layer the berries, nuts, yogurt and granola then serve.
Day 13 **Snack** Calories: 165 Protein: 9.5 g	Ingredients: 2 clementines ½ cup edamame (may be from frozen) Directions: Peel, slice and serve.
Day 13 **Lunch** *Cauliflower Mash Leftover* Time: 10 min Serves 6 Calories: 370 Protein: 25 g	Use leftovers from day 12 dinner.
Day 13 **Dinner** *Portabella Mushroom Sandwich* Time: 10 min Serves 1 Calories: 427 Protein: 13 g **Total calories: 1571** **Total protein: 57.5 g**	Ingredients: 1 portabella mushroom 1 slice of tomato 2 slices of lettuce 2 slices of whole grain bread ¼ c white wine (any kind like a Riesling or Pinot Grigio would be fine) 1 T vegan butter 1 T garlic powder 1 T onion powder 1 T vegan mayo Salt to taste

	Directions: Toast bread if desired. Saute mushroom with wine, salt, and butter for 10 minutes. Place mushroom and other ingredients between the slices of bread then close sandwich, cut in half and serve.
Day 14	
Day 14 **Breakfast** ***Crunchy Cashew Soy Yogurt*** Time: 10 min Serves 1 Calories: 568 Protein: 14 g	Ingredients: ¼ c cashews, chopped 1 cherry or strawberry soy yogurt (I like Silk or Whole Soy) 1 whole grain English muffin 2 T organic jelly or spreadable fruit Directions: Toast the muffin and spread the jelly on each half. Sprinkle the cashews over the yogurt and enjoy separately.
Day 14 **Snack** Calories: 340 Protein: 16 g	Ingredients: ½ mango 1 oz. almonds 1 c soy milk Directions: Peel, slice and serve.
Day 14 **Lunch** ***Basil Tomato Couscous*** Time: 10 min Serves 3	Ingredients: 1 c whole grain couscous 4 slices of tomato, cubed 2 leaves of fresh basil (or 1 T dry) 1 lemon ½ T garlic powder

Calories: 367 Protein: 15 g	½ c vegetable broth 1 t hot sauce Salt to taste Directions: Add all ingredients except the tomato in a pot and cook couscous in veggie broth instead of water according to package directions. Garnish with the tomato and serve.
Day 14 **Dinner** Mashed Potato and Smoked Tofu Time: 10 min Serves 2 Calories: 383 Protein: 11 g **Total calories: 1658** **Total protein: 56 g**	Ingredients: 1 block of extra firm tofu, cubed 4 potatoes, thick slices 1 package of vegan mozzarella cheese 1 c scallions, chopped 2 c green beans 2 T vegan butter 1 T vegan Worcestershire sauce 2 T garlic powder ¼ c soy sauce 1 t hot sauce 1 T black pepper Salt to taste Directions: Boil potatoes in a pot with water enough to cover potatoes for 15 minutes. Mash potatoes with a potato masher and mix with cheese and butter while still hot. Add salt to desired taste. Place 1 T of butter in a large pan over medium heat. Add several pieces

	of tofu on the pan and cook for 5 minutes. Sprinkle tofu evenly with garlic powder, soy sauce, and Worcestershire sauce then cook for additional 10 minutes turning over cubes as they brown. Serve immediately.

www.ingramcontent.com/pod-product-compliance
Lightning Source LLC
Chambersburg PA
CBHW060454280326
41933CB00014B/2748